Essential Oils

Essential Oils for beginners your guide to healing with aromatherapy and essential oil recipes for beauty and health

By

Beatrice Anahata

© **Copyright 2019- All rights reserved.**

The contents of this book may not be reproduced, duplicated or transmitted without direct written permission from the author.

Under no circumstances will any legal responsibility or blame be held against the publisher for any reparation, damages, or monetary loss due to the information herein, either directly or indirectly.

Legal Notice:

This book is copyright protected. This is only for personal use. You cannot amend, distribute, sell, use, quote or paraphrase any part or the content within this book without the consent of the author.

Disclaimer Notice:

Please note the information contained within this document is for educational and entertainment purposes only. Every attempt has been made to provide accurate, up to date and reliable complete information. No warranties of any kind are expressed or implied. Readers acknowledge that the author is not engaging in the rendering of legal, financial, medical or professional advice. The content of this book has been derived from various sources. Please consult a licensed professional before attempting any techniques outlined in this book.

By reading this document, the reader agrees that under no circumstances are is the author responsible for any losses, direct or indirect, which are incurred as a result of the use of information contained within this document, including, but not limited to, —errors, omissions, or inaccuracies.

Table of Contents

Do you like essential oils?... 6

BASIC RECIPES 8

Acne 24

Aging Skin 26

Air Freshener... 28

Anger.. 30

Anxiety 32

Arthritis 34

Asthma 36

Back Pain 39

Bathroom Care 41

Blisters 43

Bloating 45

Body Odor 46

Bronchitis 50

Bug Bites and Stings 52

Bug Repellent.. 54

Cellulite 57

Chapped Lips 60

Chilblains 62

Colds and Flu 65

Colic 68

Conjunctivitis	70
Cough	72
Cradle Cap	74
Cuts and Scrapes	75
Diaper Rash	78
Diarrhea	80
Ear Infection	82
Eczema	84
Fatigue	86
Fever	88
Flatulence	90
More Recipes	97
Conclusion	142

Do you like essential oils?

Essential oils are something that many people seem to love to try, and they have a wide variety of different uses. But, what are the best ones? What are the best ways to use them? What are the best benefits that you can get from these different oils, and how complex is it to use these invaluable oils on your body and in your home?

Obviously, they can help our body in a ton of different means, but at the same time, you might wonder what the best ones to use are, and what the best uses for these are. Well, you're about to find out.

Essential oils can typically be used either topically, in a diffuser, diluted with a carrier oil such as coconut or olive oil, or they can be used in water or other cleansers to help spray it into an area. There are so many different ways to use these and often, you probably feel overwhelmed as to what does what. Well, let's go over just what extent these essential oils can help you.

This chapter will go into detail on how you can use essential oils, including the top benefits for this. They're very simple to use, and you can get started with these right away. By using them, you'll be able to have a better home for yourself, and for others, and from there, you'll be able to create a better life for yourself too. Natural medicine can really help you out, and essential oils are definitely the way to go. You'll be able to learn about the top benefits here, and what oils you can use to accomplish these various measures to help your life.

BASIC RECIPES

We typically recommend the following:

if you are going to use a topical (a blended recipe smoothed on the body with an oil or cream, or essential oils on a compress, or "neat" for instance), always inhale it directly first. Bioavailability is better with inhalation, meaning more effective and swifter action in that route, but in many instances, topical is also useful as it works slower and lasts longer the skin. In other words, for most applications calling for a topical, it makes sense to also inhale.

INSOMNIA

- Simply diffuse lavender at night in the bedroom. Simplicity at its best. In addition, you could add a few lavender drops to your washing machine when you wash your sheets and pillowcases; you could put a few drops of lavender on a cotton ball or in a sachet and tuck it under the pillow.
- Blend 10 drops lavender, 10 drops Roman chamomile, 4 drops vetiver and 4 drops clary

sage in an ounce of carrier oil. Apply on neck, wrists and feet at night and inhale or diffuse. (I like to use the rollerball applicators in a glass bottle – easy when you are tired at night and effective.)
- Buy a premade Sleep Blend. Many companies offer them (including mine). Our Zen Sublime Sleep is blended in an organic carrier oil so it can be applied to your skin as well as inhaled or diffused. Here is the blend and why I chose each EO:

- Lavender – well known and most used essential oil for sleep assistance. Lavender calms, soothes and nurtures. It helps to balance the spirit, and reduces any existing anxiety. It also helps reduce pains which may hinder sleep.
- Rose Geranium – fosters a sense of security and protects from disturbing energy or thoughts.
- Orange – unblocks energy; found in clinical tests to be a sedative that calms, pushes down pessimism and is a tonic for mind and body.
- Neroli – relaxes nerves, soothes the heart and psyche, and helps relieve pain.

- Cedarwood – is very grounding, a tonic for the nervous system and is of course anti-inflammatory.
- Clary Sage – well-known to reduce anxiety and stress, which may be the cause of sleeplessness. It works synergistically with lavender for sedation and calming effect.

Sore Throat

- Do a steam inhalation of 2 drops Chamomile, 3 drops Lavender and 1 drop Thyme.
- For simplicity, do a steam inhalation of just 2 drops Clove.
- After a steam inhalation, massage the blend of 2 drops Lemon, 1 drop Thyme and 4 drops Chamomile in a tablespoon of a carrier oil onto your throat and neck (including behind your ears.)
- (From Aromahead) Put one drop of Tea Tree in a glass of warm water, mix it, and then gargle. Don't worry if you swallow a little, but try to spit out most of it. Gargle like this several times a day. You can also put one drop of Sandalwood in a bit of jojoba and rub it on the front and back of your neck.
- Make this blend to inhale or diffuse every 3 hours. 12 drops lavender, 6 drops black pepper and 3 drops myrrh.

- Buy a premade blend. There are many available!
- I personally find that if a sore throat is making it's appearance and hasn't really taken hold, I inhale Eucalyptus every hour (and sometimes I will also inhale myrrh and/or clove) and it goes away.

Tonsillitis

- Blend in 2 teaspoons of a carrier oil 6 drops Rose Geranium, 4 drops Myrrh and 2 drops Orange or Sweet Orange. Massage on the throat and neck, and inhale.
- Put 1 drop of Tea Tree in 1 tsp of honey plus 1 cup of warm water, mix well then gargle (do not swallow.)

Cough

- Blend 2 drops Eucalyptus, 2 drops lemon and 1 drop Tea Tree in 2 teaspoons honey. Dilute in a cup of warm water and gargle.
- For a spasmodic cough: blend 2 drops Cypress and 1 drop Frankincense on a cotton ball or tissue, inhale deeply.
- For a spasmodic cough (from Aromahead): blend 5 drops Black Pepper, 5 drops

Frankincense and 5 drops Black Spruce in a personal handheld inhaler. Use as needed.
- Dry cough: Mix Eucalyptus 3 drops, and Thyme 2 drops in 1 teaspoon of a carrier, massage on chest and throat.
- Blend Eucalyptus, Cedarwood, Pine and Myrrh in 1/6 ounce bottle. Inhale, use in a diffuser or tent steam; or mix with a carrier oil 1 ounce and massage on the throat.

Tooth Ache

- Dot Clove onto a Q-tip and touch the affected area. It will help reduce pain and inflammation.

Congestion

- Do a Eucalyptus steam. Add 10 drops of Eucalyptus and 10 drops of Siberian Fir Needle with 8 drops of Tea Tree and 2 drops Myrrh to boiling water. Make a steam tent with a towel and inhale with eyes closed.
- Put 2-4 drops of Eucalyptus in the corner of your shower in the morning, and let the steam rise and help you. Make sure to put the drops where you won't stand or step to avoid slipping.
- Blend Eucalyptus, Myrrh, Peppermint and Lemon or diffuse any one of these (your

choice) to help break up congestion and breathe better. They will also clarify the air.
- Buy a premade blend that can be massaged on your chest and throat as well as inhaled. Ours is blended in organic jojoba and sunflower and includes:
- Eucalyptus - well-known and wide ranging benefits, including sinus and respiratory applications, increases blood flow and helps with mental exhaustion. It is known to be anti-inflammatory, antispasmodic and very importantly, a decongestant.
- Rosemary - In addition decreasing the levels of cortisol (a stress hormone which can kick in when you are sick which hurts the immune system), Rosemary oil has properties believed to be helpful in relieving respiratory issues and reducing pain.
- Juniper Berry - among its many qualities, Juniper Berry is a detoxifier or purifier of blood, helping to remove toxins.
- Lime - Limes, like lemons, are full of antioxidants, bactericides and other beneficial nutrients. It helps to fight and protect against viral infections which may cause the common cold. Additionally, lime is an antiseptic, meaning it can cure infections and protect against their development.

Headache
- There are different types of headaches, from a sinus headache, migraine to a tension headache. Here are a few suggestions:
- For many types of headaches, use a cool compress or washcloth. Swish the cloth in cool water with 2 drops lavender and 1 drop peppermint, or 2 drops lavender and 1 drop Rose Geranium (inhale to see what you react to better). Put the cold compress on your forehead and relax in a darkened room.
- General headache for no reason: 3 drops Lavender and 1 drop peppermint, use neat or blend in 1 tsp of a carrier. Apply and massage around the temples, back of neck and around the hairline (be sure to patch test first any EO used neat.)
- Nervous headache: 3 drops lavender and 2 drops chamomile or an alternative is 1 drop Rose Geranium, 2 drops lemon and 3 drops lavender in 1 tsp of a carrier. Massage in and relax.
- Sinus headache: steam inhale 3 drops rosemary, 1 drop thyme and 1 drop peppermint or eucalyptus.
- Acute sinusitis: Combine 4 drops eucalyptus, lavender, peppermint, pine and tea tree in a bowl, drop in a wick for an inhaler or cotton

balls, then place inside the personal inhaler and use 5 times a day.
- Do the same recipe but only 1 drop of each in hot water and do a steam inhalation.
- In a pinch, inhale eucalyptus directly from the bottle frequently.
- Tension headache: Blend into 1 ounce of cream 3 drops lavender, 4 drops Frankincense, 1 drop Rosemary and 1 drop Helichrysum. Run on the back of your neck and temples when tension begins.
- General headache: Put 4 drops of lemon in 1 tsp of carrier, and drop in a bath and relax in the tub.
- Buy a premade blend, made by many companies.

Anxiety Attack

- Blend 10 drops each of Lavender, Geranium and Rosemary and diffuse or inhale.
- Blend Neroli 7 drops, Lavender 3 drops and Lemon 20 drops; diffuse.
- For guilt & depression that spurs anxiety: 15 drops Rose Geranium, 10 drops Bergamot, Lavender 5 drops, Turmeric 5 drops; diffuse.
- Inhale or diffuse Rosemary or Lavender alone.

Plain Old Stress
- Blend 3 drops Lavender, 3 drops Bergamot, 1 drop Rose Geranium and 1 drop Frankincense in a diffuser or personal inhaler.
- Blend 3 drops of Clary Sage, 1 drop of Lemon and 1 drop Lavender in your diffuser or personal inhaler.
- Massage Blend. Blend into 1 ounce of a carrier oil 5 drops Cedarwood, 5 drops Bergamot, 2 drops Jasmine or Ylang Ylang and 1 drop Neroli.
- Buy a premade blend. We love ours – Zen De-Stress is blended in organic jojoba and sunflower oil, and includes:
    - Lavender – lavender essential oil has the ability to eliminate nervous tension, relieve and calm. The refreshing aroma also helps with nervous exhaustion and helps lower blood pressure.
    - Clary Sage – is an anti-depressant among its many powers. It helps fight depression and relieves anxiety while helping to boost joy.
    - Neroli – is also an anti-depressant along with holding sedative powers. It helps drive away sadness and lifts the mood (which is why this oil is

extensively used in Aromatherapy techniques.)
- o Roman Chamomile – is excellent for combating stress, and helps those who are depressed, lonely or fearful. It helps calm, and is also good for times of anger or irritability.

TUMMY RUB FOR CONSTIPATION (From Aromahead)

- Blend into 1 ounce of cream 7 drops Sweet Marjoram, 3 drops Bergamot, 3 drops Orange, 2 drops Neroli, 1 drop Roman Chamomile and 5 drops Spikenard. Massage on tummy several times daily.

TUMMY RUB FOR IBS OR CRAMPS (From Aromahead)

- Blend into 2 ounces of a cream 5 drops of Orange, 5 drops Roman Chamomile, 5 drops Sandalwood and 4 drops Bergamot. Massage on belly and lower back every few hours.
- Blend 6 drops Turmeric into a carrier oil. (Add 2 drops Bergamot if desired) Massage on tummy.
- Blend 2-3 drops Clove and 4 drops Roman Chamomille into a carrier oil and massage onto your tummy. Can also help relieve gas

Bliss And Relaxation
- For an uplifting yet blissful feeling, blend into 1 ounce of cream or oil 2 drops Rose Geranium, 2 drops Bergamot, 1 drop Orange.
- Buy a premade blend. Our Zen Air Bliss contains: Ylang Ylang, Sweet Orange, Bergamot, Magnolia and Neroli.

Muscle Pain And Stiffness
- Blend into 1 ounce of a carrier like jojoba or baobab: 4 drops Eucalyptus, 4 drops Black Pepper, 4 drops Lavender and 2 drops Rosemary. Rub on the affected area as needed (every 2 hours when there is acute pain.)
- You can put the same recipe on a compress without the carrier (cool or warm). Drop the essential oils into a bowl of water (heated or cooled), swish your cloth in it, wring out and apply. For extra power, put your carrier solution on the skin; then apply the compress.

Swollen Muscles And Joints
- Blend into 1 ounce of a carrier oil 8 drops Roman Chamomile, 3 drops Lavender, 4 drops Frankincense, 3 drops Helichrysum.
- Simplicity for arthritis or rheumatoid arthritis: use Frankincense or Turmeric, or blend both in an oil or cream; twice daily, massage into

the affected joints. Diffuse Frankincense or Turmeric when desired.

Cuts

- Put 1-2 drops of Lavender neat on the cut, or
- Put 1-2 drops of Helichrysum neat on the cut, or
- Put 1-2 drops of Rose Geranium on the cut.
- Each will serve as an antibacterial and healing agent. Rose Geranium has a clotting action and helps stop the bleeding. (I keep these 3 in the kitchen for handy use.) Turmeric does the same thing, and is good as a followup for healing in a gel or cream.

Leg Cramps

- Blend 2 drops Peppermint, 4 drops Cypress, 2 drops Ginger, and 2 drops Sweet Marjoram with 4 teaspoons carrier oil of your choice and massage in.
- Blend into 15 ml of Coconut oil or other carrier oil 5 drops Rosemary oil, 3 drops Lavender oil, 2 drops Turmeric and 6 drops Marjoram oil. Massage in circular motions.
- In a pinch, simply blend Peppermint in jojoba oil and massage in.

- Check if your calcium, magnesium and potassium levels are off or not in balance. This could cause cramps, among other things.

Cold Sores
- (courtesy Aromahead.) Blend 30 drops Sandalwood and 3 drops Eucalyptus radiate into 1 ounce of aloe vera gel. Dab it on the cold sore or area where it is developing ever hour.

Acne
- Tea Tree and Juniper Berry are two essential oils that have been studied and tested with acne. Tea Tree is effective on acne and oily skin, and juniper berry is a good antibacterial for acne.
- Tea Tree could be used "neat" but do the patch test first. Simply drop 2-3 drops of Tea Tree onto the acne or pimple twice daily. Otherwise, blend into jojoba which works with well with the skin.
- Blend Tea Tree and Juniper into an aloe gel or jojoba oil, and use as a serum to tamp down oil and breakouts.

PESTS (Mice, Rats, Cockroaches)
- These pests hate or fear Peppermint. Put 4-5 drops of Peppermint on a tea bag and place at the back of kitchen cabinets or where there may be holes in the wall or cabinets (points of entry) as a deterrent. Likewise, Clove is helpful against spiders and bugs. Make sure your dog or cat can't get at the tea bag!

Refreshing Your Home

We have mentioned some uses throughout the book. Here are just a few of them:
- Put 2 drops of Lavender in your washing machine or a 1 drop on the dryer cloth when doing bed linens – or any laundry!
- Put 1 drop of Lavender in your dishwasher to help disinfect and freshen.
- Use your favorite essential oil (Lemon, Lime or Bergamot work well) to wipe down surfaces. Put drops into spray bottle with water or white vinegar.
- Use Tea Tree on a paper towel to wipe around areas that get fungi or mold (inside hidden areas of washer, drains, bathroom corners.
- Diffuse your favorite essential oils in various rooms for various situation, such as: energetic children at night – diffuse lavender an hour before bedtime (and in the

bedroom if desired). Sick ones at home – diffuse clove or eucalyptus or lemon. Want a tranquil environment – diffuse frankincense. A joyful one – do a blend like Zen Bliss, or diffuse sweet orange, ylang ylang, frankincense or bergamot. Grieving – diffuse Rose Geranium. Diffuse your favorite essential oil.
- There are hundreds more recipes and uses for essential oils, and I hope this has given you a jumping off point!

Go Wild With Wild Orange

One essential oil that is actually great for many home remedies, including nervous system issues, is wild orange. The first thing that you'll notice the second that you have this is that it smells utterly amazing, and most people love this for the smell alone. However, did you know that there are so many properties that you can use this for? Did you know that you can use it to help with inflammation, bacteria, digestive system issues, and even to help with sedation? That's right, it works for all of these, and it can definitely help you in your everyday life. You can go wild with wild orange, and it contains most of the benefits that essential oils can give to you.

It's also a means to help really kill bacteria. By diffusing a few drops into a space, it will directly kill bacteria.

Now, if you do choose to use this on the skin, wait about 6 hours before you go out into the sun since it can cause a sensitivity, and it might burn the skin.

If you want an essential oil that smells good and contains a lot of the medical benefits that you're looking for, then look no further for wild orange is ready to go and save the day. Have this, use this on the body, and from there, you can reap the benefits of this on the system, and it'll allow you to have a much better life as a result from this.

Acne

Thanks to medical science, we know that acne is a skin condition aggravated by hormonal changes in the body—and not a reaction to chocolate. Cleansing the skin properly helps those stricken with blemishes fight the production of sebum, the oily substance that clogs pores. Replicated studies in Australia and India have determined that tea tree essential oil is as effective at fighting acne (killing the specific bacteria that cause acne) as the pharmaceutical benzoyl peroxide, so you can battle a breakout with a natural, cost-effective remedy.

Neat Acne Swab

Makes 1 treatment

2 drops tea tree essential oil

1. In the morning, wash your face with mild soap and water, and dry with a clean towel.
2. Place 2 drops of tea tree essential oil on a cotton swab or cotton ball.
3. Gently dab each pimple with the cotton swab or ball.

Acne Night Treatment

Makes 10 treatments

30 drops orange essential oil

15 drops carrot seed essential oil

5 drops juniper essential oil

5 drops Roman chamomile essential oil

1. In a small glass or metal bowl, mix the orange, carrot seed, juniper, and Roman chamomile essential oils neat (undiluted), and pour the mixture into a small (5-mL) dark amber or cobalt glass bottle. Close the bottle tightly and keep it closed until you are ready to use the blend.
2. Before bed, place 5 drops of the oil blend on a cotton swab or cotton ball and rub over your acne. Leave it on for 5 minutes, then dab off any excess with a tissue.
3. Apply nightly until the acne fades. Store the remaining blend in a cool place out of direct sunlight.

Aging Skin

Excessive sun exposure, smoking, or a diet low in antioxidants can all cause skin to age sooner and more rapidly than we would like. The astringent and regenerative properties of essential oils can renew your skin and help slow the aging process. I've chosen sweet almond oil and jojoba oil for carrier oils because of their soft texture, moisturizing effects, and pleasant scents.

Aging Skin Tightening Rub

Makes 4 to 8 treatments

2 tablespoons sweet almond oil

12 drops sandalwood essential oil

8 drops geranium essential oil

1. In a small glass or metal bowl, combine the sweet almond oil with the sandalwood and geranium essential oils. Store in a 1-ounce dark amber or cobalt glass bottle.
2. After cleansing your skin, smooth 1 teaspoon of this blend onto your face and neck.
3. Use once daily. Store the remaining blend in a cool place out of direct sunlight.

Aging Skin Eye Wrinkle Defense

Makes 6 to 9 treatments

6 tablespoons jojoba oil

30 drops myrrh essential oil

1. In a 4-ounce dark amber or cobalt glass jar, combine the jojoba oil and myrrh essential oil. Cap the jar and shake well to combine.
2. Using the tip of your finger, or with a cotton swab, gently apply a few drops to the skin under your eyes and massage until the oil is absorbed.
3. Use once daily. Store the remaining blend in a cool place out of direct sunlight.

Air Freshener

How does that stale smell come into your home? If you have to keep windows closed during a long winter, you can still freshen the air indoors with essential oils. A simple mix of these oils with water will provide enough natural deodorizing power to keep you from spending money on perfumed chemical-based air fresheners.

Pine Air Freshener Spray

Makes 16 ounces

2 cups water

16 drops eucalyptus essential oil

16 drops pine essential oil

16 drops tea tree essential oil

1. In a pint-size glass or metal spray bottle, combine the water with the eucalyptus, pine, and tea tree essential oils. Cap the bottle and shake well to combine.
2. Mist this freshener around your house wherever—and whenever— it will do some good.

3. Store the remaining blend in a cool place out of direct sunlight.

NOTE: In addition to the essential oils used in this recipe, many other essential oil combinations will work, too: lemon and eucalyptus for a clean scent, or orange, clove, and sandalwood for warm, bright notes.

Anger

How often do we hear that we should step back and take a deep breath when something makes us angry? Here's a way to make that pause to breathe as effective as possible: Scent it with the calming effects of aromatherapy. These recipes will help you find the fragrances that bring you back to earth, whether you use them at home, in the car, or at the office.

Anger Diffuser Treatment

Makes 1 diffusion

3 drops chamomile (German or Roman) essential oil

3 drops balsam fir essential oil

3 drops rose essential oil

3 drops sandalwood essential oil

1. To the water in your diffuser, add the chamomile, balsam fir, rose, and sandalwood essential oils, and turn it on. Let the diffuser run for at least 15 minutes. Breathe.

Anger Spray Blend

Makes 1 ounce

2 tablespoons distilled water

3 drops lavender essential oil

1 drop clary sage essential oil

1 drop galbanum essential oil

1 drop peppermint essential oil

1. In a 1-ounce glass or metal spray bottle, combine the water with the lavender, clary sage, galbanum, and peppermint essential oils. Cap the bottle and shake well to combine.
2. Spray this blend at home, in the car, or use it (judiciously) in an area of your workplace where you can enjoy it without objection from your coworkers. If you have an office with a door, close the door before spraying.
3. Store the remaining blend in a cool place out of direct sunlight until you need it again.

Anxiety

Many essential oils can help ease the anxiousness that comes with daily work and life. The solutions suggested here can bring relaxation and release when the day's events overwhelm your sense of well-being. Milk aids the oils' absorption into the bath water, so they don't float on top.

Anxiety-Releasing Bath

Makes 1 treatment

½ cup milk

4 drops sandalwood essential oil

1 drop ylang-ylang essential oil

In a small glass or metal bowl, mix the milk with the sandalwood and ylang-ylang essential oils.

Run a warm bath and then add the milk and oils to the warm water.

Step in, breathe in the scents, and relax.

Anxiety-Reducing Spray

Makes 2 ounces

4 tablespoons distilled water

6 drops lavender essential oil

2 drops cedarwood essential oil

2 drops geranium essential oil

2 drops spearmint essential oil

1. In a 4-ounce glass or metal spray bottle, mix the water with the lavender, cedarwood, geranium, and spearmint essential oils. Cap the bottle and shake well to combine.
2. Spray 2 or 3 pumps in your home or car, as needed.
3. Store the remaining blend in a cool place out of direct sunlight. Remember to shake again before each use.

Arthritis

Wherever the pain of arthritis strikes, a topical application of essential oils with their anti-inflammatory properties can help bring relief to stiff, aching joints. Clove and sandalwood essential oils can also provide penetrating pain relief. In addition to Biblical essential oils, add evening primrose, a carrier oil that is one of nature's most effective anti-inflammatory oils. If evening primrose is not available, jojoba oil or sweet almond oil are good substitutes.

Arthritis Pain Relief Rub

Makes 6 treatments

2 tablespoons evening primrose oil

15 drops clove essential oil

15 drops sandalwood essential oil

1. In a 2-ounce dark amber or cobalt glass bottle, mix the evening primrose oil with the clove and sandalwood essential oils. Cap the bottle and shake well to combine.
2. Apply about 1 teaspoon of this mixture directly to the affected area and massage it into the skin.

3. Repeat as needed for pain. Store the remaining blend in a cool place out of direct sunlight.

Arthritis Cooling Rub

Makes 12 treatments

4 tablespoons evening primrose oil

24 drops eucalyptus essential oil

24 drops balsam fir essential oil

12 drops spearmint essential oil

1. In a 4-ounce dark amber or cobalt glass bottle, mix the evening primrose oil with the eucalyptus, balsam fir, and spearmint essential oils. Cap the bottle and shake well to combine.
2. Apply 1 teaspoon of this mixture directly to the affected area and massage it into the skin.
3. Store the remaining blend in a cool place out of direct sunlight.

Asthma

Nothing is more frightening than watching your child with asthma struggle to breathe, or to feel the restriction in your own airway. Essential oils can help relieve asthma symptoms through inhalation, especially when activated with heat. An asthma attack can be life threatening, so if using these methods does not improve breathing, use your prescription medications and seek the help of your physician or visit an emergency room, as needed. You can still use the following methods to supplement your doctor's instructions, but restoring breathing is the first priority.

Asthma Steam Relief

Makes 1 treatment

3 cups water

¼ teaspoon (25 drops) eucalyptus essential oil

1. In a small pot over high heat, heat the water until it simmers.
2. Turn off the heat and add the eucalyptus essential oil.
3. Place a trivet or hot pad on a surface you can bend your head over. Place the pot on the trivet. Cover your head with a towel and bend

over the steaming water, using the towel to trap the steam. Breathe deeply.
4. Come up for fresh air when you need it, and continue to breathe the steam until the water cools.
5. Do this as often as you like, refreshing the water with new hot water and eucalyptus essential oil.

NOTE: You can substitute lavender or peppermint essential oil for the eucalyptus.

Asthma Vapor Rub

Makes 4 treatments

- ¼ cup olive oil
- 12 drops lavender essential oil
- 8 drops geranium essential oil
- 2 drops frankincense essential oil
- 2 drops peppermint essential oil

1. In a 4-ounce dark amber or cobalt glass bottle, combine the olive oil with the lavender, geranium, frankincense, and peppermint essential oils. Cap the bottle and shake well to combine.
2. Rub about 1 tablespoon of the mixture onto the chest. This remedy is particularly effective just

before bedtime, so after application, cover up with an old t-shirt or a pajama shirt.
3. Store the remaining blend in a cool place out of direct sunlight.

Back Pain

If you know your back pain comes from the hours you spend standing at work, the new workout you took on a little too enthusiastically, or the way-too-late night you spent at the keyboard, these remedies will help loosen your muscles and take the edge off the pain. If, however, you have a ruptured disk or serious injury, see your doctor before you begin any alternative care plan.

Back Pain Rub

Makes 3 to 4 treatments

2 tablespoons olive oil

10 drops balsam poplar essential oil

10 drops rosemary essential oil

6 drops lavender essential oil

4 drops cassia essential oil

4 drops eucalyptus essential oil

1. In a small glass or metal bowl, mix the olive oil with the balsam poplar, rosemary, lavender, cassia, and eucalyptus essential oils.

2. Rub (or have someone rub) some of the blend into your sore back muscles.
3. Do this twice daily until the pain subsides. Store the remaining blend in a 1-ounce dark amber or cobalt glass bottle in a cool place out of direct sunlight.

Back Pain Soak

Makes 1 treatment

½ cup Epsom salt

10 drops clary sage essential oil

10 drops lavender essential oil

1. In a small glass or metal bowl, use a spoon to combine the Epsom salt with the clary sage and lavender essential oils.
2. Run a warm bath. Add the salt mixture to the water all at once and swish the water around to dissolve the salt.
3. Soak in the tub for 15 to 20 minutes.

Bathroom Care

If the smells of ammonia and chlorine do not appeal to you, several essential oils and odorless baking soda can change the way you clean and disinfect your bathroom.

Bathroom Grout Spray

Makes 16 ounces

2 cups water

2 teaspoons (200 drops) tea tree essential oil

1. In a pint-size glass or metal spray bottle, mix the water and tea tree essential oil. Cap the bottle and shake well to combine.
2. Spritz the mixture on grout or caulking that has mildewed. Don't rinse it—let it work away at the stains. Repeat as needed to defeat mildew and mold.
3. Store the remaining blend in a cool place out of direct sunlight.

Bathtub Cleaner

Makes 1 application

- 1 cup baking soda

- 24 drops grapefruit essential oil
- 24 drops tea tree essential oil
1. In a medium glass or metal bowl, mix the baking soda with the grapefruit and tea tree essential oils.
2. Sprinkle this powder on your tub and scrub it with a sponge or brush.
3. Rinse with water. The waxy soap buildup will rinse away.

Toilet Cleaner

Makes 20 ounces (6 to 10 uses)

- 2¼ cups water
- ¼ cup unscented liquid castile soap
- 4 drops lavender essential oil
- 4 drops lemon essential oil
- 4 drops tea tree essential oil
1. In a 32-ounce glass or metal spray bottle, combine the water, castile soap, and the lavender, lemon, and tea tree essential oils. Cap the bottle and shake well to combine.
2. Spray this in your toilet bowl and scrub it with a brush.
3. Flush to rinse. Store the remaining blend in a cool place out of direct sunlight.

Blisters

When fluid is trapped under your skin, it forms a blister, like a bubble on the surface. Blisters can be painful when they burst, and the underlying tissue can become infected. Sometimes these bubbles form as a result of herpes simplex or athlete's foot. Here's how to keep them from becoming more than a nuisance.

Blister Disinfecting Treatment

Makes 5 treatments

10 drops carrier oil of choice

5 drops benzoin (onycha) essential oil

5 drops lavender essential oil

5 drops myrtle essential oil

1. In a small (5-mL) dark amber or cobalt glass bottle, add the carrier oil followed by the benzoin, lavender, and myrtle essential oils. Cap the bottle and shake well to combine.
2. Apply about 5 drops to a cotton swab and gently pat the broken skin, getting the oil under the broken skin and in contact with the exposed layer.

3. Cover with an adhesive bandage or use a doughnut-shaped moleskin to protect the area if you need to wear shoes.
4. Apply twice daily until the blistered skin closes. Store the remaining blend in a cool place out of direct sunlight.

Blister Interim Care

Makes 1 treatment

1 to 2 drops German chamomile or frankincense essential oil

1. Once the dead skin has lifted naturally away from the blistered spot, carefully trim it off.
2. Treat the new skin underneath with 1 to 2 drops of essential oil daily until it toughens.

Bloating

The mild to severe discomfort of bloating can be a symptom of many things: general indigestion, food allergies or sensitivities, bowel obstruction, or even serious disease. Lemon essential oil acts as a natural diuretic, which can help get things moving again; coriander and peppermint have properties that relieve gas and bloating. If time and the natural remedy provided here do not relieve the situation, seek the help of your physician.

Bloating Relief Rub

Makes 1 treatment

- 6 drops olive oil
- 2 drops coriander essential oil
- 2 drops lemon essential oil
- 2 drops peppermint essential oil
1. In a small glass or metal bowl, stir together the olive oil with the coriander, lemon, and peppermint essential oils.
2. With your fingertips, apply the blend in a clockwise direction to the abdomen.
3. Lie on your left side for 15 minutes. Breathe in the scents of the essential oils to expand their effectiveness and help you relax.

Body Odor

Body odor comes from bacteria that thrive on the body when you perspire, so people who are more physically active are more likely to produce an odor. You can use body sprays and commercial deodorants to combat this, but essential oils provide a natural option that may be a better fit for your lifestyle.

Deodorant Spray

Makes 3 ounces (5 to 6 applications)

- 6 tablespoons grain alcohol
- 30 drops tea tree essential oil

1. In a 4-ounce glass or metal spray bottle, mix the alcohol with the tea tree essential oil. Cap the bottle and shake well to combine.
2. Spray this on your clean armpits after you shower. Store the remaining blend in a cool place out of direct sunlight.

NOTE: For the grain alcohol, I recommend Everclear. In addition to the tea tree essential oil used in this recipe, lavender, lemon, pine, or spearmint essential oils are also antibacterial, and will work well if you prefer one of these scents.

Deodorant Stick

Makes 1 deodorant stick

- ¼ cup aluminum-free baking soda
- ¼ cup arrowroot or cornstarch
- 5 drops of one of the following antibacterial essential oils:
- cumin essential oil
- geranium essential oil
- lavender essential oil
- lemon essential oil
- lime essential oil
- pine essential oil
- spearmint essential oil
- thyme essential oil

3 to 5 tablespoons coconut oil

1 empty stick deodorant container

1. In a small glass or metal bowl, mix the baking soda and arrow-root with the essential oil of choice.
2. One tablespoon at a time, add the coconut oil and blend with a pastry blender until fully blended into a paste consistency. Press this into your deodorant container and let stand until the coconut oil solidifies.

3. Apply as needed. Store the remaining blend in a cool place out of direct sunlight.

Deodorant Stick For Hot Climates

Makes 1 deodorant stick

- 1½ teaspoons grapeseed oil
- ¾ teaspoon shea butter
- ¾ teaspoon vegetable glycerin
- 1 tablespoon baking soda
- 3 drops cassie essential oil or absolute
- 3 drops eucalyptus essential oil
- 3 drops peppermint essential oil
- 3 drops pine essential oil
- 3 drops cistus essential oil

1. In a small glass or metal bowl, combine the grapeseed oil, shea butter, and glycerin.
2. Microwave for 10 seconds on high, or until the shea butter melts.
3. Stir in the baking soda and the cassie, eucalyptus, peppermint, pine, and cistus essential oils. Pour the mixture into an empty deodorant container.
4. Refrigerate until it solidifies, and keep refrigerated between uses.

NOTE: This deodorant is especially good for use in warm climates because the shea butter works to combat odor in high heat.

Bronchitis

When the respiratory system becomes inflamed with the respiratory disease known as bronchitis, it produces excess mucus and long spasms of coughing. Bronchitis can worsen and lead to pneumonia, and it can be an indicator of a more serious condition such as chronic obstructive pulmonary disease. Eucalyptus and rosemary are both effective at opening constricted bronchial passages, so direct treatment can be helpful. If your case does not respond to these treatments in one to two days, seek the advice of your physician.

Bronchitis Eucalyptus Diffusion

Makes 1 diffusion

5 drops eucalyptus essential oil

1. To a diffuser, add the eucalyptus essential oil. Take the diffuser into a contained space such as a closed bedroom.
2. Turn on the diffuser and let it run until all the oil has diffused.

Bronchitis Steam Treatment

Makes 1 treatment

3 cups water

¼ teaspoon (25 drops) eucalyptus or rosemary essential oil

1. In a small saucepan over high heat, heat the water to a simmer.
2. Turn off the heat and add the eucalyptus essential oil.
3. Place a trivet or a hot pad on a surface you can bend your head over. Place the pot on the trivet. Cover your head with a towel and bend over the steaming water, using the towel to trap the steam. Breathe deeply.
4. Come up for fresh air when you need it, and continue to breathe the steam until the water cools.
5. Do this as often as you like, refreshing the water with new hot water and essential oil.

Bug Bites and Stings

When mosquitoes bite and the bites become itchy, we want relief as quickly as we can get it. Essential oils with anti-itch properties can solve this problem in minutes, and they can be applied as often as necessary until the bumps disappear. Bee stings are a more serious issue—they can cause pain, fever, and even headaches, and people who are allergic to them can have more dangerous reactions. If the stinger remains in the wound, it can create greater pain and swelling. Check first with a magnifying glass and remove the stinger with tweezers, or by scraping with a credit card. When the stinger is gone, apply an essential oil that has antihistamine and anti-inflammatory properties.

Neat Bug Bite Itch Treatment

Makes 1 treatment

1 drop lavender, peppermint, or wintergreen essential oil

1. Apply 1 drop of the essential oil of choice directly on the sting every 15 minutes for the first hour after the sting. All 3 oils listed have antipruritic (anti-itch) properties, so they will ease the discomfort of the insect sting.

2. After the first hour, apply 1 drop of any one of these oils 3 times daily until the sting stops bothering you.

Bee Sting Cold Compress

Makes 1 treatment

2 cups cold water

10 drops galbanum essential oil

1 drop chamomile (German or Roman) essential oil

1. In a medium glass or metal bowl or a low basin, mix the water and galbanum essential oil.
2. Soak a hand towel in the water, allowing it to absorb the liquid.
3. Wring out the towel and place it on the bee sting. Wrap it in place using a second hand towel and plastic wrap.
4. If you can, leave this on for several hours (change the compress with a fresh one as it gets warm), and you will defeat the swelling and quell the pain.
5. Once you remove the compress, apply 1 drop of undiluted chamomile essential oil, 3 times a day, directly on the sting location.

Bug Repellent

Here you'll find information for keeping mosquitoes and other biting insects at bay. Citronella is well known as an effective mosquito repellent, and you can buy candles, lamp oil, and a number of other products that dispense it. In the first remedy below, it gets a boost from a number of nature's other effective oils. While few substances are as effective at chasing away mosquitoes as the chemical known as DEET, citronella is also scientifically proven to ward off insects, especially when mixed with pure vanilla extract (the same kind you use in baking—but make sure it's pure vanilla and not imitation). It has a shorter interval of effectiveness than DEET, however, so reapply at least every three hours.

Natural Insect Repellent

Makes 2 or 3 applications

2 tablespoons grain alcohol or rubbing alcohol

12 drops citronella essential oil

12 drops eucalyptus essential oil

6 drops cedarwood essential oil

6 drops geranium essential oil

1. In a small glass or metal bowl, mix the alcohol with the citronella, eucalyptus, cedarwood, and geranium essential oils. Stir to combine well. Transfer to a 2-ounce glass or metal spray bottle.
2. Apply sparingly to your skin, as this is highly concentrated.
3. Use as needed on clothing (except silk, which will be stained on contact) and on the brim of your hat rather than applying all over your skin.
4. Store any remaining repellent in a 1-ounce dark amber or cobalt glass bottle in a cool place out of direct sunlight until you need it again.

NOTE: For the grain alcohol, I recommend Everclear.

Citronella And Vanilla Insect Repellent

Makes 8 ounces

1 cup water

1 tablespoon pure vanilla extract

6 drops lavender essential oil

4 drops lemongrass essential oil

3 drops citronella essential oil

2 drops ginger essential oil

1. In a 12-ounce glass or metal spray bottle, combine the water with the vanilla extract and the lavender, lemongrass, citronella, and ginger essential oils. Cap the bottle and shake well to combine.
2. Spray on your skin and clothing (but not silk, which will be stained on contact), and around the brim of your hat.

Do not spray on your face.

3. Repeat as needed to deter mosquitoes. Store the remaining blend in a cool place out of direct sunlight.

Cellulite

Women tend to have more body fat than men do, and a woman's skin has a thinner outer layer than a man's skin. When the fat packets in women's skin just below the epidermis become enlarged, they become the visible "cottage cheese" skin we know as cellulite. Sadly, no method has been discovered that makes cellulite disappear, but some essential oils can help break it down and make it less visible.

Daily Cellulite Massage

Makes 8 ounces (10 to 14 treatments)

1 cup grapeseed oil

20 drops fennel essential oil

20 drops juniper essential oil

10 drops of one of the following:

- cypress essential oil
- grapefruit essential oil
- lemon essential oil
- rosemary essential oil
- sage essential oil

1. In a small glass or metal bowl, combine the grapeseed oil with the fennel and juniper essential oils, and the essential oil of choice. Mix well.
2. Before you use the massage oil, use a dry body brush (such as a sisal brush) to gently brush the cellulite-stricken areas of your body until your skin is pink.
3. Daily, massage the oil into your cellulite areas for 10 minutes to diminish its appearance.
4. Store the remaining mixture in a dark amber or cobalt glass bottle or jar in a cool place out of direct sunlight.

Cellulite Helichrysum Treatment

Makes 1 treatment

1 tablespoon olive oil

5 drops helichrysum essential oil

1. In a small glass or metal bowl, mix the olive oil and helichrysum essential oil.
2. Daily, massage this blend into your problem cellulite areas until it is absorbed into your skin and you see results.

NOTE: Helichrysum essential oil is a natural anti-inflammatory, making it effective for a wide range of skin issues. If you're not seeing the results you want from your daily massage (and you've already taken off some weight and you're getting regular exercise), try adding this to your daily regimen.

Chapped Lips

Whether you live in a climate with six months of bitter winter or in the bone-dry desert, you know what discomfort chapped lips can create. These simple remedies give you moisturizing relief along with the regenerative powers of essential oils. Which one you use is entirely a matter of personal preference; some people prefer the clear, shiny aloe vera gel on their lips, while others like the richness of shea butter.

Chapped Lips Gel

Makes 1 treatment

1 large drop aloe vera gel

1 drop frankincense or myrrh essential oil

1. Place 1 drop of aloe vera gel on your index finger.
2. Add 1 drop of your essential oil of choice.
3. Smooth between your finger and thumb to mix.
4. Apply to your lips. Repeat as often as you like to fight dryness and chapping.

Shea Butter For Chapped Lips

Makes 1 treatment

1 fingertip's worth of shea butter (about ¼ teaspoon)

1 drop cistus essential oil

1. Place the shea butter on your index finger.
2. Add 1 drop of cistus essential oil.
3. Smooth between your finger and thumb to mix.
4. Apply to your lips. Repeat as often as you like to fight dryness and chapping.

NOTE: If you don't have cistus essential oil, lavender, myrrh, or frankincense essential oil will work.

Chilblains

If you've been exposed to cold, damp conditions for long periods, you may know the discomfort of chilblains—also known as pernio. The small, swollen, itchy spots on fingers, toes, ears, and nose are not life threatening, but they can be a nuisance.

Chilblains Layering Treatment

Makes 1 treatment

1 drop myrrh essential oil

1 drop lavender essential oil

1 drop helichrysum essential oil

3 drops sweet almond oil

1. Using your fingertips, apply the myrrh essential oil to the affected area.
2. Next, apply the lavender essential oil on top of the myrrh.
3. Now apply the helichrysum essential oil over the lavender.

4. Top these with the sweet almond oil.
5. Repeat this up to 4 times daily until the chilblains are healed.

Soothing Sandalwood And Cedarwood Bath For Chilblains

Makes 5 treatments

5 tablespoons calendula oil

6 drops cedarwood essential oil

6 drops lavender essential oil

6 drops sandalwood essential oil

1. In a 4-ounce dark amber or cobalt glass bottle, combine the calendula oil with the cedarwood, lavender, and sandalwood essential oils. Cap the bottle and shake well to combine.
2. Run a warm bath and, while the water is running, add 1 tablespoon of the blend to the warm water.
3. Soak for at least 15 minutes.
4. Repeat daily until the chilblains are healed.

5. Store the remaining bath oil in a cool place out of direct sunlight.

Colds and Flu

Sneezing, sniffles, upper respiratory congestion, coughing, and low-grade fever are all common symptoms of the world's most ubiquitous and contagious malady. There's no cure for the common cold and no easy way to fight the flu, but you can arm yourself against the next onslaught by keeping some antiviral and symptom-fighting essential oils on hand, including eucalyptus, fir, frankincense, lavender, lemon, myrrh, myrtle, spearmint, and tea tree.

Cold- And Flu-Fighting Steam

Makes 1 treatment

1 to 1½ cups steaming-hot water

1 drop balsam fir essential oil

1 drop lavender essential oil

1 drop myrrh essential oil

1 drop tea tree essential oil

1. Into a medium glass or metal bowl set on a heatproof surface, pour the hot water.
2. Add the balsam fir, lavender, myrrh, and tea tree essential oils.

3. Place a trivet or hot pad on a surface you can bend your head over. Place the bowl on the trivet. Cover your head with a towel and bend over the steaming water, using the towel to trap the steam. Breathe deeply.
4. Come up for fresh air when you need it, and continue to breathe the steam until the water cools.
5. Repeat this process as often as you wish.

Vapor Rub For Colds And Flu

Makes 5 treatments

2 tablespoons sweet almond oil or jojoba oil

15 drops rosemary essential oil

10 drops eucalyptus essential oil

5 drops lemon essential oil

1. In a 2-ounce dark amber or cobalt glass bottle, combine the sweet almond oil with the rosemary, eucalyptus, and lemon essential oils.
2. Gently rub this blend on your chest, neck, cheekbones, and around your nose, following the line of your sinus cavities.

3. Repeat 2 to 3 times daily until your symptoms clear. Store the remaining blend in a cool place out of direct sunlight.

Colic

When your baby cries uncontrollably for hours at a time, and continues to cry like this more than three days a week for several weeks in a row, she has colic—and you have sleepless nights and high stress levels. The condition is not permanent, but no parent can bear to hear their baby cry without doing something to soothe her.

Colic Massage

Makes 1 treatment

1 teaspoon sweet almond oil

1 drop geranium essential oil

1 drop lavender essential oil

1. In your palm, mix the sweet almond oil with the geranium and lavender essential oils until they are warm.
2. Using a little of the oil on your fingertips, gently rub this blend in a circular, clockwise motion on your baby's stomach.
3. When the baby becomes quieter, turn him over onto his stomach and continue the gentle massage on his back.

Colic Warm Compress

Makes 1 compress

2 cups warm water

1 drop lavender essential oil

1. In a small glass or metal bowl, combine the water and lavender essential oil.
2. Place a washcloth on the surface of the water and let it become saturated.
3. Lift the washcloth from the water and wring out the excess water.
4. As your baby lies on her back, place the wet compress on her stomach. Once the compress cools to the point it no longer keeps your baby warm and comfortable, remove it.
5. If the crying begins again, repeat the process.

Conjunctivitis

Conjunctivitis, or "pink eye," is an infection of the transparent membrane covering the white part of the eye. Not only is it irritating, it's also highly contagious, and children often pass it from one to the next. You can take steps to relieve the itching and soreness using warm compresses and rose essential oil, but anything you use must be disinfected immediately to keep from spreading the infection to others in the family.

Conjunctivitis Compress

Makes 1 compress

2 cups warm water

5 drops rose essential oil

1. In a small glass or metal bowl, combine the water and rose essential oil.
2. Place a washcloth on the surface of the water and let it become saturated.
3. Lift the washcloth from the water and wring out the excess water.
4. Place the wet compress over the affected eye. (It may be easiest to have your child lie down

for this, or for you to lie down if you're the one affected.)
5. When the compress cools to the point it no longer feels warm, remove it. Immediately wash out the compress with soap and hot water, and wash your hands, as well.
6. Repeat as often as you wish. If the condition doesn't clear up in 2 to 3 days, see your doctor. The infection may be bacterial rather than viral, and antibiotics may be required.

Cough

Colds, allergies, and post-nasal drip can create a nagging tickle that just doesn't seem to go away. Cough drops made with honey or horehound can be effective natural remedies. While no essential oil should be taken internally, you can soothe the cough using your vaporizer and a range of essential oils—and throat and chest rubs can penetrate to help clear the source of the tickle.

Chest Rub For Cough

Makes 5 treatments

2 tablespoons olive oil

15 drops eucalyptus essential oil

10 drops balsam fir essential oil

1. In a 2-ounce dark amber or cobalt glass bottle or jar, combine the olive oil with the eucalyptus and balsam fir essential oils.
2. Rub this blend over your chest and throat.
3. Repeat as desired. Store the remaining blend in a cool place out of direct sunlight.

Cough Congestion-Busting Vapor

Makes 1 treatment

3 drops each of 1 or more of the following:

>chamomile essential oil (German or Roman)

>frankincense essential oil

>ginger essential oil

>lavender essential oil

>oregano essential oil

>sandalwood essential oil

>tea tree essential oil

1. To the water in your vaporizer, add the essential oils of choice, and turn it on.
2. Stay in the room with the vaporizer running for at least 15 minutes every hour.
3. Repeat as often as you wish.

Cradle Cap

It looks potentially worrisome to new parents, but cradle cap is a very common ailment that children grow out of after the age of one. The crust of dead skin cells can be remedied with a simple balm that kills bacteria when gently massaged into your baby's scalp.

Cradle Cap Scalp Treatment

Makes 1 treatment

1 teaspoon jojoba oil

2 drops geranium or rose geranium essential oil

1. In your palm, combine the jojoba oil with the geranium essential oil. Rub both palms together to warm the oils.
2. Gently apply the blend to your baby's scalp. Be careful not to get any of the oil in his eyes.
3. With a baby brush, gently rub the oil into the affected area.
4. Repeat this 3 times daily until the condition clears.

Cuts and Scrapes

Use the antiseptic and antibacterial qualities of essential oils in place of commercial first-aid creams for minor cuts and scrapes. Many essential oils can prevent infection and allow your wound to heal naturally and effectively, without the sting of an alcohol-based disinfectant.

Wash For Minor Cuts

Makes 1 treatment

Warm water

3 drops of one of the following:

      eucalyptus essential oil

      lavender essential oil

      lemon essential oil

      pine essential oil

      sandalwood essential oil

      spikenard essential oil

      tea tree essential oil

1. Fill a sink or large glass or metal bowl with warm water.
2. Add 3 drops of the essential oil of choice.
3. Bathe the cut or scrape in the water, then dry with a clean towel.

Neat Treatment For Cuts And Scrapes

Makes 1 treatment

1 or 2 drops of one of the following antibacterial essential oils:

- eucalyptus essential oil
- lavender essential oil
- lemon essential oil
- pine essential oil
- sandalwood essential oil
- spikenard essential oil
- tea tree essential oil

1. Place 1 or 2 drops of the essential oil of choice directly on the cut or scrape.
2. If there is a chance the wound could pick up dirt or could be reinjured, use sterile materials to bandage the cut or scrape.
3. Change the bandage daily, and reapply the essential oil, neat, with each new bandage.

NOTE: Eucalyptus, lavender, and tea tree essential oils are all soothing, as well as good shields against infection.

Diaper Rash

If you don't like the idea of using commercial diaper rash products on your baby's sensitive skin, essential oils provide an alternative. Here are options that will cool the rash and bring comfort to your baby.

Soothing Diaper Rash Wash

Makes 20 treatments

10 drops lavender essential oil

10 drops yarrow essential oil

2 cups warm water

1. In a small (5-mL) dark amber or cobalt glass bottle, blend the lavender and yarrow essential oils. Cap the bottle and shake well to combine.
2. In a medium glass or metal bowl, combine the water with 1 drop of the lavender-yarrow essential oil blend.
3. Soak a soft cloth in the warm water, wring it out, and use it to cleanse your baby.
4. Dry the diaper area and use a cotton ball to apply additional oil-treated water to your baby's bottom.
5. Store the remaining oil blend in a cool place out of direct sunlight until needed.

Diaper Rash Protection

Makes 20 treatments

10 drops lavender essential oil

10 drops yarrow essential oil

4 teaspoons sweet almond oil or jojoba oil

1. In a small (5-mL) dark amber or cobalt glass bottle, blend the lavender and yarrow essential oils. Cap the bottle and shake well to combine.
2. In your palm, mix the sweet almond oil with 1 drop of the lavender-yarrow essential oil blend.
3. Smooth a light layer of this protective oil over the diaper area before putting on a new diaper.
4. Store the remaining blend in a cool place out of direct sunlight until needed.

Diarrhea

The clinical definition of diarrhea includes watery bowel movements of abnormal frequency—say, every hour or so for several hours or longer. An intestinal disorder of this kind can make you pass a quart of liquid in a day, so drinking lots of water (or sports drinks that supply the electrolyte balance you need) is the most important thing you can do. Diarrhea that lasts two days or more becomes a health risk because of the danger of dehydration. If you frequently experience loose stools that you can't connect to a stomach virus or food poisoning, you may have a chronic condition that requires medical intervention. If your diarrhea does not begin to clear up after four days, consult your doctor.

Antibacterial Massage For Diarrhea

Makes 3 treatments

1 tablespoon olive oil

9 drops lavender essential oil

3 drops cedarwood essential oil

3 drops eucalyptus essential oil

3 drops tea tree essential oil

1. In a 1-ounce dark amber or cobalt glass bottle, combine the olive oil with the lavender, cedarwood, eucalyptus, and tea tree essential oils. Cap the bottle and shake well to combine.
2. Apply 1 teaspoon to your abdomen, massaging it in a circular, clockwise motion until the oils are absorbed.
3. Repeat as needed after each episode of diarrhea. Store the remaining blend in a cool place out of direct sunlight.

Ear Infection

Not every earache is an infection. Some come from a buildup of fluid in the ear, which becomes painful when the pressure increases during a cold or when seasonal allergies flare up. When pain persists even when the sinus congestion has cleared, there may be an infection present, and if the pain continues for more than a few hours, it's time to have a doctor take a look inside. Ear infections can cause long-term complications, especially in children. If you have a baby or toddler who keeps holding or pulling on one ear and you can see redness inside, call your doctor.

Ear Infection Olive Oil Remedy

Makes 4 treatments

1 tablespoon warm olive oil

2 drops cedarwood essential oil

2 drops lavender essential oil

2 drops Roman chamomile essential oil

2 drops rosemary essential oil

1. In a 1-ounce dark amber or cobalt glass bottle, mix the olive oil with the cedarwood, lavender, Roman chamomile, and rosemary essential oils. Cap the bottle and shake well to combine.
2. With a cotton swab, apply the oil around the opening of the ear, around the outside of the ear, and on the earlobe.
3. Place a warm compress (such as a folded washcloth soaked in warm water and wrung nearly dry) over the affected ear to warm the oils and help them penetrate.
4. Repeat every 2 hours until the pressure subsides. If the pain continues for more than 6 hours, consult a doctor.
5. Store the remaining blend in a cool place out of direct sunlight.

Ear Infection Cotton Remedy

Makes 1 treatment

3 drops lavender essential oil

1. Place the lavender essential oil on a cotton ball, and place this over the ear opening.
2. Leave it in place overnight.

Eczema

Eczema presents as red, itchy, peeling patches of skin that arise in a multitude of situations, from using a new soap or detergent to enduring a period of prolonged stress. When you find yourself scratching where you usually don't scratch, reach for your essential oils to calm the inflammation.

Eczema Anti-Itch Blend

Makes 3 to 5 treatments

1 tablespoon coconut oil

2 drops frankincense essential oil

2 drops helichrysum essential oil

1 drop geranium essential oil

1 drop thyme essential oil

1. In a small glass or metal bowl, mix the coconut oil with the frankincense, helichrysum, geranium, and thyme essential oils.
2. With your fingers, apply this blend to the itchy areas.
3. Cover the treated area with gauze. If the area is on your hand or foot, put on white cotton

gloves or cotton socks. Keep the area covered throughout the day. If you must remove the gauze or gloves, reapply the treatment, up to 3 times per day.
4. Repeat as needed until the itching stops.
5. Store any unused blend in a small (5-mL) dark amber or cobalt glass bottle in a cool place out of direct sunlight.

Fatigue

If you prefer to battle that 3 p.m. drowsiness with a natural remedy instead of an energy drink, your essential oils can help. The best cure for fatigue is sleep, of course, but that's not practical in the middle of the workday or if your evening is loaded with your children's activities. Here are some remedies to help you keep moving when your eyelids have other ideas.

Fatigue-Fighting Diffusion

Makes 4 diffusions

4 drops anise essential oil

4 drops cassia essential oil

3 drops cinnamon essential oil

3 drops pine essential oil

2 drops bdellium essential oil

1. In a small (5-mL) dark amber or cobalt glass bottle, mix the anise, cassia, cinnamon, pine, and bdellium essential oils. Cap the bottle and shake well to combine.
2. Add 4 drops of this blend to your diffuser, and run the diffuser for 15 minutes in your car or

office (if you have one with a door), or at home.
3. Cap the jar tightly and store any remaining oil blend in a cool place out of direct sunlight.

Stimulating Air Freshener

Makes 10 applications

3 tablespoons distilled water or spring water

3 tablespoons vodka or grain alcohol

12 drops peppermint essential oil

12 drops lemon essential oil

6 drops frankincense essential oil

1. In a 4-ounce glass or metal spray bottle, mix the water and vodka with the peppermint, lemon, and frankincense essential oils. Cap the bottle and shake well to combine.
2. Spray this in your room or car once every 2 hours, as needed. Store the remaining blend in a cool place out of direct sunlight.

NOTE: Any brand of vodka will do but for the grain alcohol, I recommend Everclear.

Fever

The symptoms caused by fever can make you miserable: dizziness, lack of appetite, alternating chills and sweating, fatigue, and muscle aches. A number of essential oils (any of the mint oils, as well as bay and cassia) can help reduce a fever through their overall cooling effects. If the ill person is a child, review the precautions of the following recipe before treating young children.

Fever-Cooling Neat Treatment

Makes 1 treatment

3 or 4 drops peppermint essential oil

1. Place the peppermint essential oil on a cotton ball.
2. Apply the oil directly to the back of the neck and the soles of the feet.
3. Repeat this every 30 minutes until the fever goes down.

CAUTIONARY NOTE: Peppermint essential oil should not be used with children under 7 years of age. If your child is 7 or older, it will need to be diluted. Dilute 1 or 2 drops of peppermint essential oil in 1 tablespoon of a carrier oil of your choice before applying it to your child's skin.

Fever-Reducing Cold Pack

Makes 1 treatment

1 cup cold water

3 drops spearmint essential oil

1 drop eucalyptus essential oil

1. In a small glass or metal bowl, mix the water with the spearmint and eucalyptus essential oils.
2. Place a hand towel or a cloth bandage on the surface of the water and let it become saturated.
3. Remove the towel and wring out any excess water.
4. Place the cold compress on the forehead. Cover it with a plastic bag or sheet of plastic wrap to contain the moisture. Hold the compress and plastic in place with a hand towel, or tie it in place with an elastic bandage, just tight enough to hold the compress.
5. When the compress warms to body temperature, replace it with another cold compress. Repeat until the fever is reduced.

Flatulence

If you feel bloated, crampy, and generally uncomfortable and you feel like you're expelling a lot of gas, you are not alone. Most people produce up to three pints of it a day, and pass gas about 14 times a day, according to colon-rectal.com. This doesn't make it socially acceptable, however, and the discomfort makes it even less pleasant. The number-one remedy for flatulence in the entire essential oils apothecary is peppermint. In addition to the following remedy, you can get peppermint hard candy or other edible drops at any convenience store or drug store.

Flatulence Peppermint Rub

Makes 1 treatment

4 to 6 drops peppermint essential oil

1. Place the peppermint essential oil in your palm and rub your hands together.
2. Then, rub your palms over your stomach and around your navel in a clockwise direction. The oil will be absorbed through your skin and will help relieve indigestion and flatulence.

Eucalyptus For Respiratory Issues

Do you have breathing issues? If the answer is yes, then let's take a look at eucalyptus. This is an essential oil that is great for any homemade cleaning, since it can be used to help diffuse the air to make it cleaner. Also, it is an expectorant, which is another benefit of this. May essential oils can be used to help clear out the sinuses, and this is no exception.

Ideally, the best way to use this is to use about 10 drops of this oil, 2 tablespoons of dish soap, and some water to your mop as you clean up the floors in your house. If you have a cold or respiratory infection, use a few drops with some coconut oil and then rub it into your chest to help with the breathing issues. This is also used in a diffuser for best results, since it can help freshen up the air in your home. Eucalyptus smells great too, and while it is pretty strong and might not be for everyone, this is a great one if you're looking to help clear out your sinuses and help with breathing.

Frankincense for the Immune System

Frankincense is probably the ultimate immune system booster, but it also can help with beautification and lowering the presence of scars. It can be used as well to help reduce the feeling of pain, and it can create a better sort of relief.

Now, one thing of note, is that this is one of the pricier oils, but it's pricier for a good reason. It's actually pricy because of how much it can actually help you, and most people swear by this one and lavender as the ultimate in essential oils. You can relieve the tension headaches that might come up with it, and you can create a very relaxing bath with this, combined with lavender. You can also use this topically to help with the appearance of blemishes and scars.

If you have a cut, put a drop of it onto there to help relieve the pain that you're in. the same thing goes for bites and stings that you have, since it'll reduce the itching that is there.

The best way to use this is to combine this with lavender, since it can create the ultimate stress reliever, and it can help take out the pain from tension reaches. Using two drops of each together can help with this.

If you're going to use this to help reduce the appearance of scars, then use a couple of drops near the area each day. It does take a little bit, but it does help with the appearance of them, since often this can be quite unseemly.

However, did you know that this can also help with the emotions many of us suffer from? If you have menstrual issues, such as PMS, or even emotional issues and anxiety, rubbing a little bit of this onto the face, or even using this as a diffuser, can ultimately help you with some of the pain you're going through. You can use this to help relieve the mental tensions, and overall, it can make a big difference in the future of your health and wellness.

This is a good one that you can use all over on the body, and it definitely can make a huge difference in your overall personal wellness as well.

Peppermint for the Respiratory and Digestive Systems

Along with lavender, peppermint is probably one of the best essential oils out here, for it showcases the benefits of the oil to the respiratory as well. However, it takes it a step further, helping with the digestive system in turn as well. How though? Well, it actually is a very powerful antioxidant, and it is one of the few oils that you can ingest without having to do too much dilution. It can also be used to help with nausea, headaches, and even energy output. It can be used topically in order to help relieve pain, just make sure you don't get it into your eyes. If you want to use a cooling spritz that can help you keep cool and rejuvenate the body, then this one is for you. just putting about 5 drops in a spray bottle made of glass can really help.

If you're suffering from nausea from either morning sickness or the flu, grab the bottle, open it, and inhale it deeply. Do make sure that you take a nice, deep breath, and this can help with that.

This is the essential oil for the respiratory and digestive system, and this as well shows the powerful benefits of essential oils, and it is one of the key oils that will help you with improving your life, your breathing, and also your overall wellness.

Tea Tree Oil for bites

Bug bites are never fun, and it can be quite hard for a person that has them. They can sting, and the problem with many of them is that it can be a problem to treat, since ultimately, you might be throwing more chemicals into there than you care to admit. However, tea tree oil is a natural means to help you get the sting out of there, but it's also an oil that's actually a must for almost all homes. Why is that?

Well, it actually is a very powerful antibacterial period, meaning it can be used in the home not only as a cleaner, but it also can be used every time you get hurt. Putting it on the skin will help to fight off the infection, but as well soothe the skin, since often it can be quite painful. For burns, this is a natural slave, and it can be used to help alleviate the pain from this.

Now, if you want to help clean up the body and such, you can put this into a homemade shampoo to help bring life to your hair. If you have any sorts of rashes from whatever it might be, put it directly onto the skin to help with reducing the itching that might be there. If you want to clean up your home, you can add a few drops of this to a cleaning spray that is natural to help kill off the various germs that might be there. It also can be put directly onto surfaces to help directly kill germs, and it's natural too so it helps.

It also can be used topically to help reduce any sorts of blemishes on the skin, especially acne and other infections. It also can be put on a wart to help reduce the size of it, and if you have lice, mix it with a shampoo to help reduce the appearance of it.

This is a good one for pretty much any ouchie, and that's one of the huge benefits to essential oils. Once you know how to use it, which is typically a simple topical application, you can certainly get the most out of this, and you'll be able to reap this benefit when you do decide to use this product.

More Recipes

Altitude Sickness

Oral—Take a capsule filled with 5 drops of lemon, and 2 drops each of frankincense, cedarwood, and peppermint 1 to 3 times daily.

Alzheimer's Disease/Dementia

Topical—Massage 6 to 8 drops of lavender to the shoulders, back, and bottoms of the feet to improve sleep quality. Apply 1 to 2 drops each of frankincense, vetiver, and rosemary to the base of the neck, crown of the head, and behind the ears, 2 to 4 times daily. Apply 8 to 10 drops of orange oil on the bottoms of the feet, 1 to 2 times daily.

Inhalation—Apply 1 drop each of rosemary and peppermint oil on palms, rub together, and cup over nose and mouth to inhale as often as needed. Alternately, place 2 to 3 drops each of rosemary and peppermint oil in boiling water and place next to individual to inhale.

Amoebic Dysentery

Oral—Take a capsule filled with 3 drops each of oregano and lemongrass and 1 drop of thyme, 1 to 3 times daily.

Topical—Apply 1 drop each of basil, fennel, copaiba and thyme to the lower abdomen, 2 to 4 times daily.

Anemia

Oral—Take one or a combination of 4 to 6 drops of German chamomile, lemon, frankincense, or helichrysum, 2 times daily.

Topical—Apply 1 to 3 drops of German chamomile, frankincense, lemon, and/or helichrysum to the bottom of the feet, 2 to 4 times daily.

Aneurysm

Topical—Mix 5 drops cistus and 1 drop each of helichrysum and cypress in equal parts carrier oil and apply to the head and back of the neck, every 2 hours.

Oral—Take 10 drops of lemon, 3 to 4 times daily.

Anger

Inhalation—Place 1 drop each of ylang ylang, orange, and German chamomile on a tissue and inhale as needed.

Topical—Massage the soles of the feet (focusing on the liver area on the outside of the right foot) with 1 drop each of ylang ylang, orange, German chamomile, and lavender, 1 to 3 times daily.

Angina

Topical—Apply 1 to 3 drops each of wintergreen, clove, goldenrod, ylang ylang, and/or helichrysum over heart area, 2 to 4 times daily.

Oral—Take 10 drops of a combination of helichrysum, clove, lemon, or orange, 1 to 3 times daily.

Ankylosing Spondylitis

Oral—Take a capsule filled with 7 drops of frankincense and 3 drops each of balsam fir and copaiba, 2 to 4 times daily. Take a capsule filled with 15 drops of lemon once daily.

Topical—Apply 2 drops each of basil, balsam fir, cypress, copaiba, and lavender to the back and hips, 1 to 3 times daily. Apply 3 to 5 drops of oregano, thyme, basil, cypress, wintergreen, marjoram, and peppermint (layered in that order, 1 at a time) to the spine and massage into back on either side of the spine, 2 times weekly.

Other—Keep the back limber by performing yoga cat-cow poses for 1 to 2 minutes immediately before bedtime.

Anxiety

Topical—Apply 1 to 3 drops of lavender and cedarwood to the base of the skull, neck, and head.

Oral—Take 1 capsule filled with 3 drops each of lavender, cedarwood, and German chamomile, 1 to 3 times daily.

Inhalation—Apply 1 to 2 drops of cedarwood and lavender to 1 palm, rub together with the other palm, and cup hands over mouth and nose to inhale as often as needed.

Apnea, Sleep

Topical—Apply 1 to 3 drops of thyme and/or black spruce to the bottoms of each big toe and the feet before retiring to bed.

Inhalation—Apply 1 drop each of black spruce and balsam fir on pillowcase before bedtime.

Appendicitis

Severe abdominal pain requires medical attention. The appendix could burst if not treated in a timely manner, which allows its contents to leak out and spreads infection throughout your abdomen.

Oral—Take a capsule filed with 3 drops each of ginger, lemon, and peppermint, and 2 drops each of basil and oregano, 2 to 4 times daily.

Topical—Apply 2 drops each of wintergreen, orange, and lemon to the arch of the right foot and near the heel.

Other—**DO NOT** massage the abdomen. Appendicitis is considered a medical emergency and professional care should be sought as soon as possible.

Arachnoid Cysts

Topical—Apply 3 drops each of frankincense, vetiver, sandalwood, and blue spruce along the entire spine and to the base of the hairline. Apply 8 to 10 drops of orange oil to the feet, 2 times daily. Apply 3 to 5 drops of oregano, thyme, basil, cypress, wintergreen, marjoram, and peppermint (layered in that order, 1 at a time) to the spine and massage into back on either side of the spine, 2 times weekly.

Oral—Take a capsule filled with 5 drops each of frankincense, vetiver, and sandalwood, 2 to 4 times daily.

Arthritis (Rheumatoid)

Topical—Apply 1 to 2 drops each of peppermint, wintergreen, frankincense, eucalyptus, and copaiba to affected area as needed (cypress and helichrysum may also be added to increase circulation to affected joints). Apply 3 to 5 drops of oregano and clove to the bottom of the feet, 2 times daily.

Oral—Take 1 capsule filled with 4 drops each of frankincense, balsam fir, and copaiba, and 1 drop of nutmeg, 2 times daily.

Arthrogryposis Multiplex Congenita (Arthrogryposis)

Topical—Create a mixture of 1 drop each of marjoram, cypress, frankincense, lavender, basil, and German chamomile in 4 teaspoons of carrier oil and massage into the affected joints/muscles up to 3 times daily.

Asperger Syndrome

Topical—Apply 1 to 3 drops of blue spruce to both sides of the neck, 1 to 3 times daily. Apply 8 to 10 drops of orange oil to the bottoms of the feet, 1 to 2 times daily. Apply 2 drops each of frankincense, vetiver, and sandalwood to the forehead and behind the ears 1 to 3 times daily. Applying a mixture of 2 drops each of lavender, ylang ylang, blue tansy, and orange to the bottoms of the feet or by gently stroking the person's head with the oils on your hand may be calming during hyperactive episodes.

Inhalation—Inhaling 1 to 2 drops of lavender may reduce anxious feelings.

Other—Many individuals with Asperger syndrome are opposed to touch and certain odors, so it may be necessary to offer them the recommended oils and allow them to choose which ones to apply.

Asthma

Topical—Apply 1 to 2 drops each of ginger, myrtle, thyme, and pine to the chest as often as needed. Apply 1 to 2 drops of oregano, peppermint, thyme, and myrtle to the bottoms of the feet, 2 to 3 times daily.

Inhalation—Apply 1 to 2 drops of lavender, ginger, or myrtle to 1 palm, rub together with other palm, cup over mouth and nose and inhale. Place 4 to 6 drops each of 1 or more of myrtle, ginger or lavender in 3 inches of hot water that is not too hot to touch with your hand and cover head with towel to inhale every 4 to 6 hours.

Atherosclerosis

Oral—Ingest 4 drops each of rosemary, juniper, lemon, and ylang ylang, 2 to 4 times daily.

Topical—Apply ylang ylang, rosemary, and/or juniper on carotid arteries and over heart, 2 to 4 times daily.

Athlete's Foot

Topical—Soak foot in Epsom salts (use coarse sea salt for diabetics) bath with melaleuca (tea tree) and lavender added directly to the salts (not the water), 2 times daily. Apply 3 to 5 drops each of oregano, lemongrass, and melaleuca (tea tree) to affected areas after soaking.

ATTENTION-DEFICIT DISORDER (ADD) Or ATTENTION-DEFICIT HYPERACTIVITY DISORDER (ADHD)

Topical—Apply 1 to 3 drops each of cedarwood, German chamomile, and lavender and/or frankincense and vetiver to the back of the neck, brain stem, and head up to 8 times daily (frankincense and vetiver increase focus, lavender and German chamomile help calm anxious feelings). Apply 3 to 5 drops of orange, 2 to 3 times daily.

Oral—Take 1 capsule filled with 2 drops each of cedarwood, lavender, and frankincense, 2 times daily.

Autism

Topical—Apply 1 drop of blue spruce to both sides of the neck, 1 to 3 times daily. Apply 8 to 10 drops of orange oil to the bottoms of the feet, 1 to 2 times daily. Apply 2 drops each of frankincense, vetiver, and sandalwood to the forehead and behind the ears, 1 to 3 times daily. Applying a mixture of 2 drops each of lavender, ylang ylang, blue tansy, and orange to the bottoms of the feet or by gently stroking the person's head with the oils on your hand may be calming during hyperactive episodes.

Inhalation—Inhaling 1 to 2 drops of lavender may reduce anxious feelings.

Other—Many individuals with autism are opposed to touch and certain odors, so it may be necessary to offer them the recommended oils and allow them to choose which ones to apply.

Autoimmune Disorder (Immune Balancing Protocol)

Oral—Take a capsule filled with 3 drops each of vetiver, frankincense, lavender and spruce, and 1 drop of clove, morning and evening. Take an additional capsule with 3 drops each of clove, oregano, lemon, cinnamon, and 1 drop of eucalyptus and melaleuca (tea tree) once midday.

Back Pain

Topical—Apply a combination of 1 to 3 drops of wintergreen, black spruce, balsam fir, copaiba, peppermint, and frankincense to affected area, 2 to 4 times daily. For muscular back pain, use 2 to 3 drops of basil and marjoram instead.

Oral—Take 1 capsule with 5 drops each of frankincense, copaiba, and balsam fir, 2 times daily.

Barrett's Esophagus

Oral—Swallow 5 drops each of lemon and ginger in water, 2 to 4 times daily.

Topical—Apply 2 drops each of frankincense, ginger, lavender, and blue tansy externally to the throat and breastbone areas, 2 to 4 times daily.

Basal Cell Carcinoma

Topical—Apply 2 to 4 drops each of sandalwood, frankincense, geranium, cinnamon, and cypress to the affected area, 3 to 5 times daily. Apply 8 to 10 drops of orange oil to the bottoms of the feet, 2 to 3 times daily. Apply more geranium and helichrysum as the area begins to heal to prevent scarring.

Oral—Take 0.018 to 0.045 ml of enriched frankincense or frankincense per pound of body weight (for example, a 150-pound person would take 2.7 to 6.75 ml daily) in 3 to 6 divided doses throughout the day with food for 21 days.

Bed Wetting (Nocturnal Urination)

Topical—Apply 3 to 5 drops of cypress mixed with carrier oil over the stomach and bladder area before going to bed.

Bell's Palsy

Topical—Apply 1 drop each of frankincense, helichrysum, geranium, blue spruce, and copaiba directly behind and underneath both ears and on the affected area of the face, 2 to 3 times daily. Apply 3 to 5 drops of oregano, thyme, basil, cypress, wintergreen, marjoram, and peppermint (layered in that order, 1 at a time) to the spine and massage into back on either side of the spine, 2 times weekly.

Oral—Take 1 capsule filled with 2 drops each of clove, oregano, lemon, cinnamon, and 1 drop of eucalyptus, 2 to 3 times daily.

Benign Motor Neuron Disorder

Topical—Apply 3 to 5 drops of oregano, thyme, basil, cypress, wintergreen, marjoram, and peppermint (layered in that order, 1 at a time) to the spine and massage into back on either side of the spine, 2 to 4 times weekly; apply 1 drop each of blue spruce, vetiver, frankincense, and sandalwood behind the ears and at the base of the skull, 2 to 4 times daily. Apply 10 drops of orange oil on the bottoms of the feet, 2 times daily. Apply 1 to 2 drops each of marjoram, pine, lavender, and lemongrass to the major muscles, 1 to 3 times daily.

Oral—Take a capsule filled with 5 drops each of frankincense, sandalwood, and myrrh, 1 to 3 times daily.

Benign Prostatic Hyperplasia (Bph), Enlarged Prostate

Topical—Apply 1 drop of frankincense, myrrh, orange, balsam fir, and copaiba heavily diluted to the area between the anus and scrotum, 2 times daily.

Retention—Mix 3 drops each of frankincense, myrrh, and tsuga in 1 tablespoon of vegetable oil and insert rectally. Retain as long as possible.

Oral—Take a capsule filled with 4 drops each of oregano, vetiver, and rosemary, 1 to 3 times daily.

Bipolar Disorder

Only use in conjunction with Western medical options and with approval from a physician.

Topical—Apply 1 drop each of frankincense, cedarwood, sandalwood, spruce, and lavender to the base of the skull and behind the ears, 2 to 4 times daily. Apply 2 to 3 drops of helichrysum over the liver, 1 to 3 times daily. Apply 5 drops of orange and 2 drops of lemon to the bottoms of the feet, 3 times daily.

Oral—Take a capsule filled with 5 drops of helichrysum, 1 to 3 times daily.

Bites (Animal)

Topical—Apply 1 drop each of thyme, oregano, lavender, German chamomile, and lemongrass every 15 minutes for the first 2 hours, and then 1 time per hour for the next 24 to 48 hours. Apply peppermint to the bite as needed for pain.

Oral—Take a capsule filled with 3 drops of oregano, and 1 drop each of eucalyptus, melaleuca (tea tree), and thyme, 2 to 3 times daily.

Bladder Infection

Oral—Take 1 capsule filled with 2 drops each of clove, oregano, lemon, cinnamon, and 1 drop of eucalyptus, 2 to 3 times daily.

Topical—Apply 2 drops each of clove, oregano, eucalyptus, and cinnamon to the bottoms of the feet, 2 to 3 times daily. Apply 3 drops each of juniper, oregano, and frankincense with 10 drops of vegetable oil to the pelvic area, 1 to 3 times daily.

Other—Drink 2 8-ounce glasses of unsweetened cranberry or blueberry juice daily for 3 to 5 days.

Bleeding

Seek medical attention immediately if the blood spurts from the wound, or if it will not stop bleeding after 10 minutes of direct pressure.

Topical—Apply 1 to 2 drops of geranium, cypress, helichrysum, or lavender near the wound every 5 minutes until bleeding stops.

Other—Apply direct pressure to the wound.

Blisters

Topical—Apply 1 to 3 drops of lavender, German Chamomile, myrrh, or helichrysum to the blister several times daily.

Blisters (Fever)

Topical—Apply 1 drop of melaleuca (tea tree), clove, or rosemary to the blister several times daily.

Bloating

Oral—Take 1 to 3 drops of peppermint, juniper, and/or fennel in a capsule, 2 times daily.

Blood Clot

Abnormal blood clots can be a medical emergency and lead to a stroke, heart attack, or other serious conditions. Only use this protocol in conjunction with

Western medical options and with approval from a physician.

Topical—Massage 4 drops of lavender to the bottoms of the feet up to 3 times daily. Apply 1 to 3 drops of cistus, lemon, orange, and helichrysum to the affected area, 3 to 5 times daily.

Oral—Take 2 capsules with 3 drops each of cistus, helichrysum, orange, grapefruit, and lemon, 2 times daily.

Boils

Topical—Apply 1 to 2 drops of lavender, frankincense, myrrh, peppermint, or melaleuca (tea tree), several times daily.

Bone Spurs

Topical—Apply 1 drop each of eucalyptus, myrtle, pine, lavender, tsuga, oregano, and peppermint to affected area, 2 to 3 times daily. Alternately, apply 2 to 5 drops of wintergreen, balsam fir, or cypress to affected area, 2 to 4 times daily.

Brain Injury

Only use this protocol in conjunction with Western medical options and with approval from a physician.

Topical—Apply 1 to 2 drops each of frankincense, vetiver, cedarwood, sandalwood, and helichrysum to the base of the skull and back of the neck, 3 to 5 times daily. Apply 2 drops each of black spruce, blue tansy, and frankincense to the bottom of the feet, 2 to 3 times daily. When the person recovers enough, apply 3 to 5 drops of oregano, thyme, basil, cypress, wintergreen, marjoram, and peppermint (layered in that order, 1 at a time) to the spine and massage into back on either side of the spine, 2 times weekly.

Oral—Take a capsule filled with 3 drops each of frankincense, vetiver, sandalwood, cedarwood, and helichrysum, 1 to 3 times daily. Alternately, place 1 drop of each oil on the tongue, 1 to 3 times daily.

Brittle Bones

Topical—Apply 1 to 3 drops of wintergreen, helichrysum, and balsam fir to affected bones, 2 to 3 times daily. Women apply 1 to 3 drops of clary sage to the forehead or carotid arteries, 3 times daily. Men apply 3 drops of blue spruce to the feet, 3 times daily.

Broken Bones

Broken bones require more than essential oils. Seek medical attention to have the bone set and casted. This protocol is intended to help relieve pain and encourage normal healing of bones. It should be followed for the duration that the cast is on, applying oils for 3 weeks before resting 1 week, then repeating the application process.

Topical—Apply 3 drops each of balsam fir, cypress, helichrysum, lemongrass, and wintergreen to the area, 2 to 4 times daily.

Oral—Take a capsule filled with 5 drops each of balsam fir, copaiba, and frankincense, 1 to 3 times daily.

Other—Do not move the person if at all possible; this could make the injury worse. Apply a splint above and below the fracture sites if you are trained how to do so.

Bronchitis

Topical—Apply 3 to 5 drops of eucalyptus, ginger, myrtle, and/or copaiba to the chest as needed. Apply 3 to 5 drops each of oregano and 1 drop of thyme to the bottoms of the feet, 2 to 4 times daily.

Inhalation—Place 2 to 3 drops each of eucalyptus, myrtle, and copaiba in half cup of hot water in bowl, cover head and bowl with towel and inhale 3 to 6 times daily. To improve outcome, hold your breath for as long as possible during the inhalation then breathe out slowly.

Oral—Take 1 capsule filled with 3 drops carrier oil and 2 drops each of clove, cinnamon, lemon, oregano, and rosemary, 1 to 3 times daily.

Brucellosis

Oral—Take a capsule filled with 3 drops each of cinnamon, lemon, peppermint, marjoram, and 1 drop of nutmeg, 1 to 3 times daily.

Topical—Apply 3 drops each of lemon and peppermint to the spine as needed for fever. Apply 1 to 2 drops each of basil, marjoram, and ginger to sore muscles as needed.

Bruise/Bumps

Topical—Apply 2 to 4 drops of helichrysum, blue tansy, lavender, and/or frankincense to the bruise and surrounding area, several times daily (it is best to begin application directly after a blow that may cause a bruise).

Bunions

Topical—Apply 1 to 2 drops of lemon, wintergreen, and pine to the bunion, several times daily.

Burns

Other—Cool the area in cold water for several minutes. Do not use ice.

Topical—Apply 2 to 3 drops of lavender, melaleuca (tea tree), or German chamomile to the burn every 15 minutes until pain subsides, and then apply every two hours or as necessary until healing is complete.

Bursitis

Topical—Apply 2 to 4 drops each of wintergreen, balsam fir, and cypress to affected area, 3 to 5 times daily.

Calcific Tendinitis

Topical—Apply 2 drops each of cypress, balsam fir, eucalyptus, and wintergreen and 1 drop each of grapefruit, lemongrass, and lemon to and widely around the affected area, 2 to 3 times daily.

Oral—For difficult calcification, take a capsule filled with 8 drops of lemon, 2 drops each of frankincense and balsam fir, and 1 drop of wintergreen, 1 to 2 times daily.

Calluses

Topical—Apply 1 to 2 drops of oregano, lavender, or frankincense to the area, 2 to 3 times daily.

Cancer (Enriched Frankincense, And Disclaimer)

Both H.K. Lin, PhD, and Mahmoud Suhail, MD—who have extensive experience working with frankincense and cancer—recommend using "enriched" **Boswellia sacra** for cancer. Enriched frankincense is simply frankincense bottles that have been left open to allow the lighter chemical compounds to evaporate out, leaving the heavier chemical compounds. The bottle is allowed to evaporate until only 20 percent of the oil remains. According to Dr. Lin, this makes **Boswellia sacra** 10 times more potent. Because cancer is a devastating disease, aggressive action is often necessary to correct it. Large oral doses are frequently suggested and may be difficult to take immediately; therefore, it is prudent to work up to the recommended dosage to allow the body to adjust.

You may start with 1 quarter of the dosage, then work to half, and then to the full dose over a period of several days to a couple weeks. The same applies for orange oil when indicated. The average essential oil contains from 20 to 40 drops of essential oil per 1 mL. This figure can be used as a guide for dosing, but oils vary significantly based on their specific gravity, so it is not perfect. In general, 30 drops per milliliter is a good average.

<u>Disclaimer</u>: *Cancer is one of the most common life-threatening illnesses that affects up to half of us during our lifetime. You should never attempt to treat it alone. Ideally you will work closely with your physician and determine the best course of action that will lead you to healing. This partnership provides the greatest possibility of successful treatment and survival.*

Cancer (Bladder)

Oral—Take 0.018 to 0.045 ml of enriched frankincense or frankincense per pound of body weight (for example, a 150-pound person would take 2.7 to 6.75 ml daily) in 3 to 6 divided doses throughout the day with food for 21 days, then rest for 7 days, and restart regimen if necessary. Take a capsule with 15 drops of orange oil, 3 to 6 times daily. Take an additional capsule with 10 drops of sandalwood oil, 2 times daily.

Other—Intermittent fasting (only consuming water) for 24 hours, 2 times weekly, or 48 hours once weekly. Alternately, some practitioners recommend fasting for

30-plus days drinking only vegetable and fruit juices. Make sure they don't have added sugar.

Topical—Apply 3 to 5 drops each of sandalwood, basil, and orange to the affected area up to 6 times daily.

Cancer (Bone)

Oral—Take 0.018 to 0.045 ml of enriched frankincense or frankincense per pound of body weight (for example, a 150-pound person would take 2.7 to 6.75 ml daily) in 3 to 6 divided doses throughout the day with food for 21 days, then rest for 7 days, and restart regimen if necessary. Take a capsule with 15 drops of orange oil, 3 to 6 times daily. Take an additional capsule with 10 drops of clove oil, 2 times daily.

Other—Intermittent fasting (only consuming water) for 24 hours, 2 times weekly, or 48 hours once weekly. Alternately, some practitioners recommend fasting for 30-plus days drinking only vegetable and fruit juices. Make sure they don't have added sugar.

Topical—Apply 3 to 5 drops each of clove, tsuga, and frankincense over the bladder area up to 6 times daily.

Cancer (Brain)

Topical—Apply 1 to 3 drops each of lemongrass, lemon, oregano, German chamomile, and thyme to the base of the skull and behind the ears, 3 to 6 times daily.

Oral—Take 0.018 to 0.045 ml of enriched frankincense or frankincense per pound of body weight (for example, a 150-pound person would take 2.7 to 6.75 ml daily) in 3 to 6 divided doses throughout the day with food for 21 days, then rest for 7 days, and restart regimen if necessary. Take 0.02 to 0.067 ml (about 3 to 10 ml for a 150-pound person) of orange per pound of body weight in 3 divided doses with food daily for 21 days, then rest for 7 days, and restart regimen if necessary.

Other—Intermittent fasting (only consuming water) for 24 hours, 2 times weekly, or 48 hours once weekly. Alternately, some practitioners recommend fasting for 30-plus days drinking only vegetable and fruit juices. Make sure they don't have added sugar.

Cancer (Breast)

Topical—Rub copious amounts of frankincense, sandalwood, myrrh, blue spruce, and myrtle on breasts, several times daily.

Oral—Take 0.018 to 0.045 ml of enriched frankincense or frankincense per pound of body weight (for example, a 150-pound person would take 2.7 to 6.75 ml daily) in 3 to 6 divided doses throughout the day with food for 21 days, then rest for 7 days, and restart regimen if necessary. Take 0.02 to 0.067 ml (about 3 to 10 ml for a 150-pound person) of orange per pound of body weight in 3 divided doses with food daily for 21 days, then rest for 7 days, and restart regimen if necessary.

Other—Intermittent fasting (only consuming water) for 24 hours, 2 times weekly, or 48 hours once weekly. Alternately, some practitioners recommend fasting for 30-plus days drinking only vegetable and fruit juices. Make sure they don't have added sugar.

Cancer (Cervical)

Topical—Apply copious amounts of frankincense and tsuga over the pubic area, several times daily.

Oral—Take 0.018 to 0.045 ml of enriched frankincense or frankincense per pound of body weight (for example, a 150-pound person would take 2.7 to 6.75 ml daily) in 3 to 6 divided doses throughout the day with food for 21 days, then rest for 7 days, and restart regimen if necessary. Take 0.02 to 0.067 ml (about 3 to 10 ml for a 150-pound person) of orange per pound of body weight in 3 divided doses with food daily for 21 days, then rest for 7 days, and restart regimen if necessary.

Retention—Consider inserting 15 drops of frankincense and 5 drops of tsuga mixed with 1 tablespoon of carrier oil into the vagina on a tampon.

Other—Intermittent fasting (only consuming water) for 24 hours, 2 times weekly, or 48 hours once weekly. Alternately, some practitioners recommend fasting for 30-plus days drinking only vegetable and fruit juices. Make sure they don't have added sugar.

Cancer (Colon)

Topical—Apply copious amounts of frankincense and sandalwood over the lower abdomen, several times daily.

Oral—Take 0.018 to 0.045 ml of enriched frankincense or frankincense per pound of body weight (for example, a 150-pound person would take 2.7 to 6.75 ml daily) in 3 to 6 divided doses throughout the day with food for 21 days, then rest for 7 days, and restart regimen if necessary. Take 0.02 to 0.067 ml (about 3 to 10 ml for a 150-pound person) of orange per pound of body weight in 3 divided doses with food daily for 21 days, then rest for 7 days, and restart regimen if necessary.

Retention—Consider inserting 10 drops each of frankincense and sandalwood mixed with 30 to 50 drops of carrier oil into the rectum and retaining.

Other—Intermittent fasting (only consuming water) for 24 hours, 2 times weekly, or 48 hours once weekly; alternately, some practitioners recommend fasting for 30-plus days drinking only vegetable and fruit juices. Make sure they don't have added sugar.

Cancer (Gastric, Stomach)

Topical—Apply copious amounts of frankincense and sandalwood over the lower abdomen, several times daily.

Oral—Take 1 capsule filled with 5 to 10 drops of each listed oil—frankincense, clove, rosemary, ginger, and 2 drops of nutmeg—3 times daily for 21 days, then rest for 7 days, and restart regimen if necessary. Take 1 capsule with 5 drops each of lemongrass, basil, and cinnamon, once daily. Take 0.02 to 0.067 ml (about 3 to 10 ml for a 150-pound person) of orange per pound of body weight in 3 divided doses with food daily. If stomach irritation occurs, apply the oils topically over the stomach instead.

Other—Intermittent fasting (only consuming water) for 24 hours, 2 times weekly, or 48 hours once weekly. Alternately, some practitioners recommend fasting for

30-plus days drinking only vegetable and fruit juices. Make sure they don't have added sugar.

Cancer (Lung)

Topical—Apply copious amounts of frankincense, myrrh, and orange to the front and back of the ribs several times daily.

Oral—Take 0.018 to 0.045 ml of enriched frankincense or frankincense per pound of body weight (for example, a 150-pound person would take 2.7 to 6.75 ml daily) in 3 to 6 divided doses throughout the day with food for 21 days, then rest for 7 days, and restart regimen if necessary. Take 0.02 to 0.067 ml (about 3 to 10 ml for a 150-pound person) of orange per pound of body weight in 3 divided doses with food daily for 21 days, then rest for 7 days, and restart regimen if necessary.

Inhalation—Place 15 drops each of myrtle and eucalyptus in 3 inches of hot water that is not too hot to touch with your hand and cover head with towel to inhale every 2 hours.

Other—Intermittent fasting (only consuming water) for 24 hours, 2 times weekly, or 48 hours once weekly. Alternately, some practitioners recommend fasting for 30-plus days drinking only vegetable and fruit juices. Make sure they don't have added sugar.

Cancer (Oral)

Oral—First thing in the morning and on an empty stomach, add 2 drops each of clove, oregano, thyme and frankincense to 1 tablespoon of coconut oil; hold this mixture in the mouth and agitate regularly for 10 to 15 minutes—or until the oil thickens—then spit out (**DO NOT SWALLOW** as this procedure may pull toxins from the oral cavity). Repeat this procedure up to 3 times daily on an empty stomach. Take 0.018 to 0.045 ml of enriched frankincense or frankincense per pound of body weight (for example, a 150-pound person would take 2.7 to 6.75 ml daily) in 3 to 6 divided doses throughout the day with food for 21 days, then rest for 7 days and restart regimen if necessary; take 0.02 to 0.067 ml (about 3 to 10 ml for a 150-pound person) of orange per pound of body weight in 3 divided doses with food daily for 21 days, then rest for 7 days, and restart regimen if necessary.

Other—Intermittent fasting (only consuming water) for 24 hours, 2 times weekly, or 48 hours once weekly; alternately, some practitioners recommend fasting for 30-plus days drinking only vegetable and fruit juices. Make sure they don't have added sugar.

Cancer (Ovarian)

Topical—Heavily dilute and apply 2 to 4 drops each of thyme, sandalwood, frankincense, geranium, and cypress to the lower abdominal region area, 3 to 5 times daily.

Oral—Take 0.018 to 0.045 ml of enriched frankincense or frankincense per pound of body weight (for example, a 150-pound person would take 2.7 to 6.75 ml daily) in 3 to 6 divided doses throughout the day with food for 21 days, then rest for 7 days, and restart regimen if necessary. Take 0.02 to 0.067 ml (about 3 to 10 ml for a 150-pound person) of orange per pound of body weight in 3 divided doses with food daily for 21 days, then rest for 7 days, and restart regimen if necessary.

Other—Intermittent fasting (only consuming water) for 24 hours, 2 times weekly or 48 hours once weekly. Alternately, some practitioners recommend fasting for 30-plus days drinking only vegetable and fruit juices. Make sure they don't have added sugar.

Cancer (Pancreatic)

Topical—Apply copious amounts of frankincense, myrrh, and orange to the middle part of the left side of the back several times daily.

Oral—Take 0.018 to 0.045 ml of enriched frankincense or frankincense per pound of body weight (for example, a 150-pound person would take 2.7 to 6.75 ml daily) in 3 to 6 divided doses throughout the day with food for 21 days, then rest for 7 days, and restart regimen if necessary. Take 0.02 to 0.067 ml (about 3 to 10 ml for a 150-pound person) of orange per pound of body weight in 3 divided doses with food daily for 21 days, then rest for 7 days, and restart regimen if necessary.

Other—Intermittent fasting (only consuming water) for 24 hours, 2 times weekly, or 48 hours once weekly. Alternately, some practitioners recommend fasting for 30-plus days drinking only vegetable and fruit juices. Make sure they don't have added sugar.

Cancer (Prostate)

Topical—Apply copious amounts of frankincense, sandalwood, and myrrh over the lower abdomen several times daily.

Oral—Take 0.018 to 0.045 ml of enriched frankincense or frankincense per pound of body weight (for example, a 150-pound person would take 2.7 to 6.75 ml daily) in 3 to 6 divided doses throughout the day with food for 21 days, then rest for 7 days, and restart regimen if necessary. Take .067 ml (about 10 ml for a 150-pound person) of orange per pound of body weight in 3 divided doses with food daily for 21 days, then rest for 7 days, and restart regimen if necessary.

Retention—Consider inserting 10 drops each of frankincense and sandalwood mixed with 1 tablespoon drops of carrier oil into the rectum and retaining.

Other—Intermittent fasting (only consuming water) for 24 hours, 2 times weekly, or 48 hours once weekly. Alternately, some practitioners recommend fasting for 30-plus days drinking only vegetable and fruit juices. Make sure they don't have added sugar.

Cancer (Skin)

Topical—Apply copious amounts of frankincense, melaleuca (tea tree), and 1 of the following: balsam fir or sandalwood to affected area several times daily

Oral—Take 0.018 to 0.045 ml of enriched frankincense or frankincense per pound of body weight (for example a 150-pound person would take 2.7 to 6.75 ml daily) in 3 to 6 divided doses throughout the day with food for 21 days, then rest for 7 days, and restart regimen if necessary. Take .067 ml (about 10 ml for a 150-pound person) of orange per pound of body weight in 3 divided doses with food daily for 21 days, then rest for 7 days, and restart regimen if necessary.

Other—Intermittent fasting (only consuming water) for 24 hours, 2 times weekly, or 48 hours once weekly. Alternately, some practitioners recommend fasting for 30-plus days drinking only vegetable and fruit juices. Make sure they don't have added sugar.

Cancer (Testicular)

Topical—Mix 10 drops each of frankincense and blue spruce in 2 teaspoons of carrier oil and apply to the testicles, 2 times daily.

Oral—Take 0.018 to 0.045 ml of enriched frankincense or frankincense per pound of body weight (for example, a 150-pound person would take 2.7 to 6.75 ml daily) in 3 to 6 divided doses throughout the day with food for 21 days, then rest for 7 days, and restart regimen if necessary. Take 0.02 to 0.067 ml (about 3 to 10 ml for a 150-pound person) of orange per pound of body weight in 3 divided doses with food daily for 21 days, then rest for 7 days, and restart regimen if necessary.

Other—Intermittent fasting (only consuming water) for 24 hours, 2 times weekly, or 48 hours once weekly. Alternately, some practitioners recommend fasting for

30-plus days drinking only vegetable and fruit juices. Make sure they don't have added sugar.

Cancer (Thyroid)

Topical—Apply 1 drop each of frankincense, balsam fir, myrtle, German chamomile, and nutmeg to the neck over the thyroid, 3 to 6 times daily.

Oral—Take 0.018 to 0.045 ml of enriched frankincense or frankincense per pound of body weight (for example, a 150-pound person would take 2.7 to 6.75 ml daily) in 3 to 6 divided doses throughout the day with food for 21 days, then rest for 7 days, and restart regimen if necessary. Take 0.02 to 0.067 ml (about 3 to 10 ml for a 150-pound person) of orange per pound of body weight in 3 divided doses with food daily for 21 days, then rest for 7 days, and restart regimen if necessary.

Other—Intermittent fasting (only consuming water) for 24 hours, 2 times weekly, or 48 hours once weekly. Alternately, some practitioners recommend fasting for 30-plus days drinking only vegetable and fruit juices. Make sure they don't have added sugar.

Cancer (Uterine)

Topical—Heavily dilute and apply 2 to 4 drops each of thyme, sandalwood, frankincense, geranium, and cypress to the lower abdominal region area, 3 to 5 times daily.

Oral—Take 0.018 to 0.045 ml of enriched frankincense or frankincense per pound of body weight (for example, a 150-pound person would take 2.7 to 6.75 ml daily) in 3 to 6 divided doses throughout the day with food for 21 days, then rest for 7 days, and restart regimen if necessary. Take 0.02 to 0.067 ml (about 3 to 10 ml for a 150-pound person) of orange per pound of body weight in 3 divided doses with food daily for 21 days, then rest for 7 days, and restart regimen if necessary.

Other—Intermittent fasting (only consuming water) for 24 hours, 2 times weekly or 48 hours once weekly. Alternately, some practitioners recommend fasting for 30-plus days drinking only vegetable and fruit juices. Make sure they don't have added sugar.

Cancer (Vaginal, Vulvar)

Topical—Heavily dilute and apply 2 to 4 drops each of sandalwood, frankincense, geranium, and cypress to the vulva and labia area, 3 to 5 times daily. Apply 8 to 10 drops of orange oil to the bottoms of the feet, 2 to 3 times daily. Apply more geranium and helichrysum as the area begins to heal to prevent scarring.

Oral—Take 0.018 to 0.045 ml of enriched frankincense or frankincense per pound of body weight (for example, a 150-pound person would take 2.7 to 6.75 ml daily) in 3 to 6 divided doses throughout the day with food for 21 days.

Other—Intermittent fasting (only consuming water) for 24 hours, 2 times weekly, or 48 hours once weekly. Alternately, some practitioners recommend fasting for 30-plus days drinking only vegetable and fruit juices. Make sure they don't have added sugar.

Candida

Topical—Apply 1 to 3 drops each of lemongrass, clove, eucalyptus, lavender, and melaleuca (tea tree) to the bottoms of the feet, 2 times daily.

Oral—Take 3 drops each of oregano, lemongrass, lavender, and lemon in a capsule, 3 times daily.

Canker Sores

Topical—Apply 1 drop of 1 or more of clove, lemon, melaleuca (tea tree), and/or peppermint directly to the canker sore several times daily. Rotating which oils are used will increase effectiveness.

Carpal Tunnel Syndrome

Topical—Apply a combination of lemongrass, marjoram, peppermint, cypress, and wintergreen to affected area, several times daily.

Oral—For added support, take a capsule filled with 4 drops each of frankincense, copaiba, balsam fir, and lemongrass, 2 to 3 times daily.

Cataracts

Topical—Apply lemongrass, frankincense, and lavender mixed with a little carrier oil widely around the orbit of the eye at night before going to bed.

Oral—Take 1 capsule filled with 5 drops each of frankincense, lavender, and lemongrass, 2 times daily.

Cavities

See your dentist to repair the cavity.

Topical—Apply clove and cinnamon oil to tooth (may require dilution), 3 times daily.

Celiac Disease

Oral—Take a capsule filled with 4 drops of lemon, and ginger, and 1 drop each of cinnamon, grapefruit, fennel, and peppermint, 3 times daily, preferably before each meal.

Cellulitis

Topical—Apply 1 drop each of helichrysum, lavender, melaleuca (tea tree), eucalyptus, and thyme to the affected area, 2 to 3 times daily.

Chapped Skin

Topical—Apply 2 to 3 drops of lavender and/or myrrh and German chamomile to affected area as often as needed.

Charcot Foot (Neuropathic Arthropathy)

Topical—Apply 8 to 10 drops of orange oil to the bottoms of the feet, 2 times daily. Massage 4 drops each of blue spruce, cypress, balsam fir, and vetiver to the top of the feet, 2 to 4 times daily. For wounds, apply 1 to 2 drops each of frankincense, copaiba, cedarwood, and lavender to the wound, several times daily.

Cherry Angioma

Topical—Apply a few drops of a mixture containing equal portions of frankincense, cistus, lemongrass, German chamomile, lavender, and orange in 4 teaspoons of carrier oil to the affected area, several times daily.

Oral —Take a capsule filled with 5 drops each of frankincense, lemongrass, and orange, 2 to 3 times daily.

Chicken Pox

Topical—Mix 5 drops each of melaleuca (tea tree), lavender, lemongrass, and German chamomile with equal parts carrier oil and apply to spots, 3 times daily.

Oral—Take a capsule with 3 drops each of lemongrass, oregano, and lemon, 2 to 3 times daily.

Chilblains

Topical—Apply 1 drop each of German chamomile, lavender, and cypress to the affected area, 1 to 3 times daily. Alternately, add 1 drop of each to each application of lotion.

Cholera

Oral—Take a capsule filled with 3 drops each of oregano and cinnamon, and 1 drop each of eucalyptus, melaleuca (tea tree), and thyme up to 4 times daily.

Other—Drink plenty of water with electrolytes to replenish what has been lost through diarrhea.

Chronic Fatigue

Topical—Apply frankincense, sandalwood, and cedarwood to the base of the skull, brain stem, and head, 2 to 4 times daily.

Inhalation—Place 2 drops of peppermint in 1 palm, rub together with other palm, and cup over nose and mouth to inhale as often as necessary.

Oral—Take a capsule filled with 3 drops each of lemongrass, myrrh, and German chamomile, 2 times daily.

Chronic Obstructive Pulmonary Disease (Copd)

Topical—Apply 3 to 5 drops of eucalyptus, myrtle, cedarwood, peppermint and/or copaiba to the chest as needed. Apply 3 to 5 drops each of oregano and 1 drop of thyme to the bottoms of the feet, 2 to 4 times daily.

Inhalation—Place 1 to 2 drops of eucalyptus, rosemary, myrtle, and peppermint in 3 inches of hot water that is not too hot to touch with your hand, and cover head with towel to inhale, 1 or 2 times daily.

Oral—Take 1 capsule filled with 2 drops each of pine, orange, lemon, eucalyptus, and ginger up to 3 times daily.

Circulation, Poor

Topical—Apply 1 to 2 drops each of cypress, helichrysum, and cedarwood to the area of poor circulation, 3 to 5 times daily.

Oral—Take a capsule filled with 3 drops each of lemongrass, cypress, clove, and cinnamon, morning and evening.

Diabetes

Topical—Apply 1 to 3 drops each of cinnamon, lemongrass, fennel, and copaiba to the bottoms of the feet, particularly the pancreas VitaFlex point on the outer edge of the left foot about midway down, 2 to 4 times daily.

Oral—Take 1 capsule with 2 drops each of cinnamon, fennel, lemongrass, and grapefruit, morning and evening.

Diarrhea

Oral—Take a capsule with 3 drops each of peppermint and fennel, 1 to 3 times daily, or until diarrhea is relieved.

Topical—Apply 1 to 3 drops of peppermint and fennel over the abdomen every hour or until diarrhea is relieved.

Other—Drink plenty of water to replenish lost fluids.

Distal Renal Tubular Acidosis

Oral—Take a capsule filled with 7 drops of lemon and 3 drops of juniper, 2 to 3 times daily.

Topical—Apply 2 to 3 drops of pine over the kidney area on the back, 3 times daily.

Diverticulitis

Oral—Take 1 capsule filled with 2 drops each of oregano, peppermint, nutmeg, cypress, fennel, and marjoram, 2 to 3 times daily.

Topical—Apply oregano, peppermint, nutmeg, cypress, fennel, and marjoram over the abdomen, 2 to 3 times daily.

Dizziness

Inhalation—Place 1 drop each of peppermint and cypress in 1 palm, rub together with other palm, and cup hands over mouth and nose to inhale as often as necessary.

Topical—Apply peppermint, frankincense, or cypress to the temples, back of the neck and shoulders.

Dopamine Deficiency

Topical—Apply 1 to 2 drops of geranium, eucalyptus, and clary sage behind and underneath the ears, 1 to 3 times daily.

Inhalation—Place 1 drop of geranium, lemon, and clary sage on a tissue and inhale as needed. Refresh tissue up to 3 times daily.

Dry Skin

Topical—Apply lavender, myrrh, or German chamomile to affected area as often as needed.

Dupuytren's Contracture

Topical—Massage 1 drop each of cistus, basil, marjoram, vetiver, and frankincense to the affected area several times daily.

Dysesthesia (Cutaneous)

Topical—Apply 1 drops each of vetiver, blue spruce, peppermint, juniper, German chamomile, and helichrysum to the area, 2 to 4 times daily.

Oral—Take a capsule with 5 drops of helichrysum and 2 drops each of vetiver, copaiba, and lavender, 1 to 3 times daily.

Dysentery

Seek medical attention if symptoms are severe or last longer than a few days.

Oral—Take 1 capsule with 4 drops each of peppermint, lemon, and oregano, 2 to 3 times daily.

Topical—Apply 1 to 3 drops of peppermint, wintergreen, fennel, or oregano to abdomen, 2 to 3 times daily.

Ear Infection

Topical—Apply 1 to 2 drops each of lavender and melaleuca (tea tree) around the ear and on the fleshy part of the ear every 30 minutes until pain subsides, and then apply every 2 hours. Apply 1 to 2 drops each of oregano, cinnamon, clove, rosemary, and lemon to the bottom of the feet every 30 minutes until pain subsides, and then every 2 to 4 hours for the next 24 hours.

Other—Apply 1 drop of melaleuca (tea tree) to a cotton ball and place inside ear, refresh every 30 minutes until pain diminishes, and then refresh every 2 hours; leave a fresh cotton ball in overnight.

Ear Mites

Topical—Apply 2 to 3 drops each of eucalyptus and melaleuca (tea tree) around the ear and on the fleshy part of the ear, 3 to 5 times daily.

Other—Apply 1 drop of melaleuca (tea tree) and eucalyptus to a cotton ball and place inside ear, and then refresh every hour; leave a fresh cotton ball in overnight.

Earache

Topical—Apply 1 to 2 drops each of peppermint and lavender around the ear and on the fleshy part of the ear every 30 minutes until pain subsides, and then apply every 2 hours. Apply 1 to 2 drops each of oregano, cinnamon, clove, rosemary or melaleuca (tea tree), and lemon to the bottom of the feet every 30 minutes until pain subsides, and then every 2 to 4 hours for the next 24 hours.

Other—Apply 1 drop of melaleuca (tea tree) to a cotton ball and place inside ear, refresh every 30 minutes until pain diminishes, and then refresh every 2 hours; leave a fresh cotton ball in overnight.

Conclusion

Essential oils have a numerous amount of benefits and they can certainly help you if you're looking to take care of some physical issues.

They can help with bodily issues, issues with beauty, and if you're sick, this can be the go-to item to help you out. They are certainly worth the money, and it's definitely something you should try to get into.

For many people, having essential oils can help to change your life. If you're worried about what your body might do with essential oils, always make sure to diffuse it. It's best that you don't ingest them unless you know for a fact that it is safe to do so. But, if you want to get into using these you can try new means in order to accomplish various tasks with them. There are so many uses, probably hundreds of them, and they can be a great way to engage in preventative medicine. You also can use them around your home, and it will get your place smelling pretty great too.

www.ingramcontent.com/pod-product-compliance
Lightning Source LLC
Chambersburg PA
CBHW052052070526
44584CB00017B/2148